The *Later* *Years*

The *Later Years*

Sir Peter Thornton KC

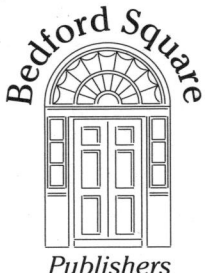

Bedford Square Publishers

First published in the UK in 2025
by Bedford Square Publishers Ltd, London, UK

bedfordsquarepublishers.co.uk
@bedsqpublishers
info@bedfordsquarepublishers.co.uk

Authorised EU representative: MustamäeTee 50, 10621 Tallin, Estonia

Copyright © Sir Peter Thornton KC, 2025

The right of Sir Peter Thornton KC to be identified as the
author of this work has been asserted in accordance with
the Copyright, Designs and Patents Act 1988.

All rights reserved. No part of this book may be reproduced, stored in
or introduced into a retrieval system, or transmitted, in any form
or by any means (electronic, mechanical, photocopying, recording
or otherwise) without the written permission of the publishers.

Any person who does any unauthorised act in relation to this publication
may be liable to criminal prosecution and civil claims for damages.

A CIP catalogue record for this book is available from the British Library.

Trade Paperback ISBN 978 1 83501 209 3
eBook ISBN 978 1 83501 210 9

10 9 8 7 6 5 4 3 2

Designed by Nicky Barneby, BARNEBY *design & art direction*
Typeset in 11.5/14.75pt Monotype Plantin by BARNEBY *design & art direction*

Printed and bound in Great Britain by Clays Ltd, Elcograf S.p.A.

For Suzie, Dan and Amy (the home team)

Disclaimer

While all reasonable care has been taken to ensure that the contents of this publication are both correct and accurate at the time of going to press, no responsibility for loss or damage occasioned to any person acting or refraining from action as a result of any statement in it (including any errors and omissions however caused) can be accepted by the author, editor or publisher. Nor should anything in this work be taken as a substitute for advice from an appropriate competent professional; if expert advice is needed, whether on health, money, wills or any other subject in this book, it should be sought.

Contents

Introduction 1

CHAPTER 1
Before Death 7
Step 1: Create a Death File 10
Step 2: Consider Your Wishes for the Future 12
Step 3: Make a Will 13
Step 4: Make an Advance Decision 19
Step 5: Make an Advance Statement 30
Step 6: Lasting Powers of Attorney 31
Step 7: Plan for Inheritance Tax 40
Step 8: Plan for Your Funeral 40
Step 9: Write a Short History 41
Mental Capacity 43
Top Ten Tips 52

CHAPTER 2
Money 53
Organise and Plan 54
Taking Advice 62
Income 65
Borrowing Money 70
Outgoings 78
Banking 85
Marriage and Civil Partnership: the Financial Advantages ... 92
Problems and Complaints 95
Treat Yourself 98
Top Ten Tips 100

CHAPTER 3
Pensions and Pension Credit — 101

The State Pension	102
Pension Credit	110
Workplace Pensions	115
Personal Pensions	118
Pension Guidance	123
Pension Complaints	123
A Pensions Dashboard?	124
Top Ten Tips	126

CHAPTER 4
Inheritance Tax — 127

Summary of IHT Rules	128
How to Calculate IHT	134
Payment of IHT	135
Further Guidance	137
Tax Planning	138
Future Changes to IHT?	140
Top Ten Tips	144

CHAPTER 5
Scams — 145

How to Avoid Fraud	145
Different Types of Fraud	147
What Do You Do When You Think You May Be a Victim?	173
The Cost of Fraud	177
Top Ten Tips	179

CHAPTER 6
Health — 180

Physical Activity	182
Mental Activity	185
Diet	186
Alcohol	190
Smoking	194
Sleep	194

Wellbeing ... 196
Dementia ... 198
Grieving ... 205
Top Ten Tips ... 207

CHAPTER 7
Home ... 208

Security Measures ... 209
Warning Alarms ... 212
Medical Aid Systems, AI ... 215
Remaining at Home by Adapting It ... 215
Accommodation Options ... 220
Sheltered Housing ... 222
Prepare for a Care Home or Nursing Home ... 225
Top Ten Tips ... 226

CHAPTER 8
Care ... 227

Home Care: Visiting Carers ... 228
Care in a Care Home ... 236
State Funding for Social Care ... 238
Recent History of Reform Proposals ... 242

CHAPTER 9
Rights ... 248

Why We Need a Charter of Rights for Older Persons ... 249
International Standards ... 250
The United Kingdom ... 253
Commissioners for Older People ... 254
A Charter of Rights ... 257
Other Important Rights ... 258
Age Discrimination ... 262
The Public Sector Equality Duty ... 265
Ageism and Discrimination ... 266
The Right to Vote ... 269
The Right to Die? ... 270
A Society for All Ages ... 270

CHAPTER 10
After Death   271

A Reminder for Those Preparing for the End of Life 271
For those who will be left behind 273
Step 1: Obtain the *Medical Certificate of Cause of Death* 275
Step 2: Register the Death 275
Step 3: Obtain Documents from the Registrar 276
Step 4: Inform Government Departments 277
Step 5: Instruct a Funeral Director 277
Step 6: Inform Relatives and Friends 282
Step 7: Place Notice of Death in the Press (if required) 282
Step 8: Plan for the Funeral (and wake) 282
Step 9: Obtain Probate 286
Step 10: Dispose of Small Personal Possessions 288
Death Referred to the Coroner 290
Top Ten Tips 292

Afterword **295**

Appendix **297**

Notes **305**

Acknowledgements **335**

About the Author **337**

Introduction

Grow old along with me!
The best is yet to be,
The last of life,
for which the first was made

Robert Browning, *Rabbi Ben Ezra* (1864)

'I always meant to, I just never got round to it'. More than half of all adults haven't made a will.[1] That is a big mistake, as you'll see when you read on.

As we know, it's not just wills. There is quite a bit more that gets left undone. For a start there are lasting powers of attorney, advance decisions and advance statements (**see pp 19–31**). And that is just the beginning.

This book, therefore, is a practical manual designed to point you in the right direction. It is not my aim to admonish you for not having planned as much as you might, but rather to look gently at the steps you could still take as an older person to ease your peace of mind and make things easier for those left behind after your death.

And this book is a good fit for me too, in my mid-seventies. Not just wills and all of that. There is much more that might just help. A little planning on money (Chapter 2), pensions (Chapter 3) and inheritance tax (Chapter 4). For example, the advantages and disadvantages of the two types of equity release; how the state pension works, where to get help on pensions, and how not to miss out on pension credit (many do); understanding the so-called nil-rate and residence nil-rate bands for inheritance tax.

And in later chapters, how to identify and avoid scams, especially those targeted at older persons (Chapter 5); the best ways to manage your ageing health (Chapter 6); how to stay at home for as long as possible (Chapter 7); and how to get the best out of care services when you need support (Chapter 8).

I also propose a Charter of Rights for Older Persons, to protect dignity and independence (Chapter 9). And finally, for those left behind after a death, there is a ten-point checklist of what to do at a difficult time (Chapter 10).

This book is for those who haven't planned, or not enough, and for their children, friends and others who may have to step up and make decisions on their behalf.

This is definitely the age of older persons. Nearly one in five of the population of the UK is 65 years or older, some 13 million people, almost double the number from the 1970s. That proportion of older people is projected to be one in four by 2050.[2]

Many of us are, of course, living longer – there are over 15,000 centenarians in England and Wales alone (more women than men).[3] Some people work later in life. Some volunteer or provide support for others, such as very elderly parents, partners or grandchildren. Other factors come into play, too. There are improvements in diet, lifestyle and healthcare. There is less smoking and improved working conditions in industry.

You don't have to look far for active older person role models. Those in their seventies, eighties and nineties (at the time of writing) in the arts, business and politics are showing the way[4]:

- Mick Jagger, Paul McCartney and Shirley Bassey are all performing; as too are Eric Clapton, Rod Stewart and Elton John
- David Hare and Tom Stoppard are writing plays; Helen Mirren, Ian McKellen and Patrick Stewart are performing in them
- David Hockney, Peter Blake and Maggi Hambling are painting, and she is sculpting too

- Norman Foster, the architect, will help Ukraine's physical reconstruction
- Richard Branson and James Dyson are still creatively active in business
- David Attenborough, Michael Palin and John Humphrys are still broadcasting
- In law, Heather Hallett chairs the UK Covid-19 Inquiry
- And you only have to look across the Atlantic to see the two older candidates for US President in 2020 (and almost, but not quite, in 2024)

But not all of us can remain active all of the time. Sometimes incapacity strikes quickly, as with an unexpected stroke or heart attack. I am suggesting in this book that you may want to be prepared. We are all likely to suffer some form of condition, disease or impairment in our later years, which will set us back temporarily or, worse, permanently. Older people are sometimes disparagingly and unfairly referred to as a 'burden' on NHS and care services. But this age group certainly presents a significant cost. It is estimated that 75% of 75-year-olds in the UK have more than one long-term medical condition, rising to 82% for 85-year-olds.[5] As somebody once said, 'I can cut the mustard. I just need help opening the jar'.

I do not dwell too much on the downsides of older age. My purpose is more positive. As Shirley Bassey once said, 'You don't get older, you get better'. I want to cherish the idea of living longer, to value and respect our generation, and help and support those who need guidance and assistance as life becomes a little more difficult. My aim, therefore, is to provide encouragement and constructive information for all of us older persons, as well as those in the generation below, all who need to plan (gently) for the more demanding times that may lie ahead.

I use the phrase 'older persons' because it identifies older people as individuals, each with his or her own wants and needs, not just a group. I may from time to time use the phrases 'older people', 'the elderly' or 'people of older age', but I have at the forefront of my mind each separate person. I mean no disrespect in any terminology I use.

'Older persons' is a phrase that is often used, sometimes in formal documents. In 1995 the United Nations Committee for the Economic, Social and Cultural Rights of Older Persons opted for this term over others including 'the aged', 'the ageing' and 'the elderly'. And 'older persons' had been used earlier by the UN General Assembly in 1991 when it adopted the UN Principles for Older Persons. No mention of 'older people' is made in either document.

It may seem a little random, but I choose 65 years as the transition from middle age to older age. Despite the fact that the state pension age in the UK has crept up to 66 (for men and women),[6] 65 is still considered to be a standard starting age for older persons. It is recognised as such by the United Nations, the World Health Organisation, the NHS and the UK's Office for National Statistics.[7]

For many, though, age is just a number; you are only as old as you feel. So, in John Welcome's 1959 novel *Stop at Nothing*, the hero complains at 40 that it's 'the first year you really feel the rot setting in and the timbers beginning to creak ... after your fortieth birthday you suddenly realise you are mortal'.[8] Or maybe 50 is old? Back in 1875, Disraeli's Government defined old age as 'any age after 50'.[9] And Victor Hugo said that '40 is the old age of youth; 50 the youth of old age.' 64? For the young Beatles, old age, 'many years from now', meant 'when I'm 64'. But in the UK, 65 is currently known as the conventional start of old age.[10] No doubt, this will advance to 70 in due course.

This book is therefore both for older people who might need a bit of help and for younger people who will be doing the helping. As Michael Caine, acting the part of an elderly composer in Paolo Sorrentino's film *Youth*, said, 'I've become old and I don't know how I got here.' We all need to prepare for that time.

This is a book for the whole of the United Kingdom, although the emphasis falls inevitably on England, by far the largest of the four nations, and Wales which shares much law with England. Where appropriate I shall highlight some of the differences in practice in Scotland and Northern Ireland.

Most chapters will end with my suggested top ten tips. These are my tips for this introduction.

Top Ten Tips

1. **Make the most of your later years** (whatever your circumstances). The UK Census shows that the 65–75 age group reports higher levels of happiness than any other age group.

2. **Be positive in everything you do.** Life expectancy is increasing; older years are becoming a greater segment of our lives.

3. **Prepare for a later working life.** With the State Pension now set at 66, working up to 65 or later is becoming more common – be prepared to adjust if necessary.

4. **Be prepared for the likely possibility of more difficult times.** Plan for the future and the possibility of less capacity (mental and physical – *see pp 43–51*); think about a will, Lasting Power of Attorneys, etc.

5. **Think about how you are going to live and manage your home.** Be prepared to adapt your home, downsize or move to a more suitable home.

6. **Stay as healthy as you can**, both physically and mentally

7. **Do a little financial planning** so that you can have greater control over your money

8. **Write a little memoir** both to reflect and to remind future generations of your family history and details of family members who might otherwise be forgotten

9. **Be a little bit organised in your life** to make things easier for loved ones when they are left behind

10. **Stand up for your rights.** You deserve respect and dignity at all times; there should be a Charter of Rights for Older Persons.

CHAPTER 1

Before Death

Prepare for death. Even though it is not an event which will take place more than once, it is better to be prepared.

Seneca, *How to die*[1]

You may be fit and healthy and live for another twenty years or more, with all your marbles intact. You may not. No one knows what the future may bring. You may suffer dementia or lose mental capacity in some other way, from a stroke or other disabling illness or injury. If you do lose the ability to make your own decisions, you may need others to make decisions for you – about health and care, money and property, where you live or how you are looked after.

These decisions may be just around the corner or they may not. Who knows? Just in case, it is time to make a few decisions of your own, while you can. Think what you would want for yourself in difficult times. Do not say, 'It may never happen to me.' **Express your wishes now**. Decide now who you can rely on to act for you later.

And help those who will want to help you. Think of your partner, family, carers and healthcare professionals. They will all want to know your wishes if and when you are unable to express them yourself.

When you die, your loved ones will have much to do as there are ten essential steps they will need to take, all during a time of grieving (*see p 274*). There is much you can do to ease that process.

This chapter helps you to think about your wishes. It encourages you to plan for the future and get organised. It advises you to put your documents and information in order and record your wishes clearly. Consider making a will, an advance decision, an advance statement and a lasting power of attorney – these could be key to your future, and they will help others.

Prepare for life, when you can no longer make decisions. And prepare, in advance, for death.

The question of mental capacity – the ability to make your own decisions – has several interesting and legal aspects to it and I go into these later in this chapter. While you still have mental capacity there are nine **practical steps** that you can take.

Nine Practical Steps:
to Complete Before Death

1	Create a death file: collect important information
2	Consider your wishes for the future
3	Make a will
4	Make an Advance Decision (living will or ADRT)
5	Make an Advance Statement
6	Make a Lasting Power of Attorney (LPA)
7	Plan for inheritance tax
8	Plan for your funeral
9	Write a short history of your life and family

This is quite a long list and a bit daunting. You could take it slowly, one at a time. A will is a must and a Lasting Power of Attorney is pretty essential. Take legal, financial or medical advice if you want to. Discuss your wishes for your future if you can. Close relatives should be grateful to know your wishes and understand what may have to be done when the time comes.

Step 1: Create a Death File

There is a lot to be said for creating a file marked with words such as ON DEATH or AFTER DEATH. This file should contain important information for the benefit of those who will be left behind. Put as many of the following as you can into the file (don't worry if you can't find them all).

The whereabouts of this file should be known by your next of kin, your nearest relative, who you can trust. Create this file now. Keep it updated. Keep it safe.

The details will be of immense value to your family when you die. Instant access to all that information, particularly at a time of great family stress, will be invaluable. It will save them time and effort in searching through your papers. It will help, for example, when the death has to be registered and when probate has to be applied for. For example, the Registrar will want to have, if available, the NHS card, birth and marriage certificates and as much relevant personal information as possible (*see pp 275-276*).

The last item will guide them through the necessary steps after death.

Old and young, we are all on our last cruise.

Robert Louis Stevenson,
Virginibus Puerisque (1881)

Contents of ON DEATH file

1. A copy of your will
2. Birth certificate; marriage certificate
3. NHS card, NHS number
4. GP contact details
5. Contact details of any other professional, probate solicitor, accountant, financial adviser
6. Family and dependants: details (names, addresses etc)
7. Financial Summary File (*see p 58*), including
   - NI and tax reference numbers
   - Details of accountant; financial adviser
   - Bank details
   - Insurance policies
   - List of income, savings
   - List of regular outgoings, debts
   - Property details
   - Other assets, including car
8. Any Advance Decision; Advance Statement
9. Any registered Lasting Power of Attorney
10. Your wishes for burial or cremation
11. Your other wishes (if any) for the funeral
12. Any other reasonable wishes
13. A short history of your life and family
14. Digital information: usernames and passwords (or where to find them)
15. A copy of the key points in Chapter 10 (*see p 272*)

Step 2: Consider Your Wishes for the Future

If you are an older person and have mental capacity (the ability) to make decisions, sit down and consider what decisions you might like to make in the future were you to lose mental capacity. Hopefully that will never happen, but it is always a possibility, for example from a stroke or from developing dementia. For the meaning of mental capacity, *see pp 43-51*.

You may want to give some thought to what you would wish for in those unfortunate circumstances. Where would you wish to live? Who would you wish to look after you? Who would you like to make decisions for you, on your healthcare and on financial matters? Any particular personal tastes? What sort of funeral service would you like? These are just a few of the questions you might like to ask yourself and discuss with those who are close to you. Having done that, you may wish to record them in writing, in the appropriate documents.

Steps 3-6 will guide you through those documents

- a will
- an Advance Decision
- an Advance Statement
- a Lasting Power of Attorney

You do not have to take any of these steps; they are your choice, although a will is definitely a must. But you should consider the alternatives. If you do not set out your wishes, others will make decisions for you and you may or may not like them. Think what you would prefer.

I loved you, so I drew these tides of men into my hands and wrote my will across the sky in stars.

T E Lawrence, *Seven Pillars of Wisdom* (1926)

Step 3: Make a Will

A will is a must. It is vitally important to make a will (although not necessarily 'across the sky in stars') so that your loved ones may carry out **your wishes**. If you do not leave a will, your wishes may positively *not* be carried out.

What is a will?

A will is a legally binding document, written, signed and witnessed, which sets out your wishes for inheritance. It details who gets what when you die. Your will sets out how your estate (property, money and personal possessions) will be distributed after your death. It also appoints executors to administer the estate according to your wishes. If there is no will, the next of kin must apply to the court to be appointed administrator of the estate (*see p 288*).

It is much easier for your loved ones if you leave a will behind. Many people, perhaps more than half of all adults, do not make a will. Many say, 'I just haven't got round to it.' But for clarity, for the future and for your peace of mind, make a will now.

Intestacy

If there is no will, you are described as dying 'intestate'. Don't die intestate. First and foremost, the consequence of intestacy is that your wishes will go unheard. Instead, the state, not you, will decide who inherits.

A will makes clear your intentions. Intestacy does not. Your family will have all sorts of expectations as to what they may inherit, but often, under the intestacy rules, they will be wrong. This can be difficult for those left behind, and sometimes appear unfair.

For example, if you are a couple living together, but are neither married nor in a civil partnership, your partner could lose out badly. You may wish to leave your house or savings to your partner. You may expect that if you die intestate your partner will automatically inherit them. But you would be wrong.

Your partner may receive nothing if there is no will. They may have been your co-habiting partner for 20 years, you may be devoted to each other, but they may get nothing. The law on wills does not recognise that relationship, a loving one but not a legal one, unless you leave a will.

In Scotland, if there is no will, it may be necessary to apply to the Sheriff Court for an executor to be appointed.[2]

There may, therefore, be real dangers of unexpected, and un-wished for, consequences if you die without a will. Where there's a will there is definitely a way forward that makes sense for you and for others.

Write a clear will

It is much better for you (and your peace of mind) and all concerned if your intentions are made clear by a **properly drafted and witnessed will**. It does not have to be a particularly formal document. But to be valid a will must be:

- in writing
- signed by you
- witnessed in your presence by two witnesses (both over 18) who will not benefit from the will
- with named executors

And you must have mental capacity and not be pressured into making it. Mental capacity to make (and sign) a will is known in the law as 'testamentary capacity'. It is broadly similar to the test of mental capacity in the Mental Capacity Act 2005 (*see pp 43–51*), although there are a few differences.[3]

You could write the will yourself. It may, however, be better to take proper advice and have your will drafted by a solicitor or professional will writer. Some banks and building societies draft wills too. Making a will with professional help does not have to be an elaborate or expensive process.

Contents of the will

A will is your opportunity to express your wishes for passing on (subject to inheritance tax) your personal estate: your **property, finances** and **personal possessions**.

You can provide **bequests** (also known as legacies) of cash to individuals (such as grandchildren) or organisations. You can make donations to charities. Most charities are exempt from having to pay inheritance tax on a gift in a will (*see p 133*). If you wish to make a charitable donation, you can sign up to the National Free Wills Network scheme; some 900 solicitors provide free will-writing services to supporters of nearly 250 specific charities: see nationalfreewills.net.

If you want to be specific about certain **items of property**, you can make a specific bequest in the will to a named person. You can ask your solicitor to make an annex to the will, listing specific items of property such as pictures or jewellery or items of sentimental value, and who they should go to. Or, if they have not been clearly included in the will, you can make specific wishes separately, preferably in writing.

And you can add into your will, if you wish, any of the following specific **arrangements for your funeral**:

- whether you wish to be buried or cremated and where
- where you would like your ashes to be scattered (if cremated)
- who you would like to arrange the funeral
- the type of funeral service
- the music to be played or poems or readings to be read
- the speakers or readers
- whether a donation to a nominated charity should be requested instead of flowers

*I owe much; I have nothing;
I give the rest to the poor.*

Francois Rabelais, *Last will* (1553)

You can also state in your will the **arrangements for your pets**. Funeral arrangements and arrangements for pets are not legally binding, even in a will, but at least it makes your wishes known.

It is better to discuss these kinds of arrangements with close relatives first. Instead of including them in your will, you could write a letter to the family or to the executors of your will. Or you could express your wishes in an Advance Statement (*see pp 30-31*).

Some people also add into their will after the words 'all my personal chattels' the words 'and all my **digital assets** (including information)'. Digital assets include photos, emails, documents stored online, any blog or website, Facebook, Instagram and other social media accounts and any money you may have left with PayPal or eBay, for example.[4]

Facebook and Instagram (both Meta), for example, will memorialise the account on request, by keeping it as a place for family and friends to share memories. Or they will permanently delete it on request. Both require proof of death. You can plan in advance for deletion of your Facebook account by saying so on the memorialisation settings page. To close an account, PayPal will require information from the executor or administrator of the estate of the deceased person.[5]

Some websites offer a service for storage of all your **passwords** until death, at which point they will be given to a named person. On the other hand, there is no such thing as absolute security online. Information of that kind, kept in a so-called 'electronic safe deposit box', could be a hacker's paradise. It might be better just to tell someone close what your passwords are (or where you keep them). They could, perhaps, be kept in your Death File (*see pp 10-11*).

You can imagine how much more difficult it will be for this information to be accessed or deleted if you die intestate. It may be sufficient to provide a copy of the death certificate and proof of next of kin. It may not. Don't die intestate. Make a will.

If you are **a couple**, whether married or in a civil partnership or neither, a will should make your intentions clear. A common form of will is a so-called *mirror will* (or *mutual will*) in which each partner leaves everything to the surviving partner, and, if there are children, to the children equally thereafter.

In your will you should also nominate, with their agreement, **executors** who will oversee the administration of your estate according to your wishes.

You may wish to be careful what you write in your will. After probate is granted (*see pp 286–288*), anyone can search probate records and apply for a copy (for a modest fee).[6] In Scotland, see mygov.scot for *Finding a will*.

Executors

Your will must name your executors, that is, those who will administer the estate after your death. They will go through the process known as 'probate'. Probate is the gathering together of your assets, the payment of inheritance tax, the payment of your debts and the distribution of the remainder to those specified in the will, in that order. For probate, *see pp 286–288*.

You can name one or more executors in your will, up to a maximum of four. An executor is usually a close relative or close friend – particularly someone you feel you can trust and who is likely to outlive you. Or an executor may be a named solicitor (or a named firm of solicitors), preferably one who is expert in dealing with wills and probate, especially where the estate is large or complex. It does not have to be any of those. It can be anyone you choose. You should ask their permission before naming them in the will.

Two executors is a good number, one professional (a solicitor) and one close relative or friend. Obtaining probate can be a difficult process. It helps, too, where a solicitor is named, to have a close relative named as well so that the solicitor has a good link person from the family to communicate with. The solicitor's fee is taken out of the estate.

An executor may benefit under a will. An executor may witness a will, but only if they are not a beneficiary.

Changing or updating a will

You can update your will by making a 'codicil'. This is a formal written document setting out your intentions. It can add to or amend the instructions in your will. A codicil must be signed and witnessed as with a will. You can make as many codicils as you wish.

Or you can replace the first will by a second. This option is better where you are making major changes.

Revoking a will

A will can be revoked by you, either by deliberate destruction or by being replaced by a later will. A fresh will should at least be considered after major changes in your life, such as getting married or divorced, having a child, or if the named executor dies.

In any event, getting married (or entering a civil partnership) nullifies a pre-marriage will, unless it was made 'in contemplation of marriage'. You must make a new will as the pre-marriage will is no longer valid.

If you get a divorce, any appointment in your will of your ex-spouse automatically lapses, as does any provision in your will to benefit them.

Challenging a will

A will can be invalid on a number of grounds. If you are worried when you discover a late change of will, for example, by your aged parent who may at the time have lacked capacity, leaving a large sum of money to a 'carer' or 'friend', you can **enter a 'caveat'** which prevents the executor (who could be the same person as the carer or friend) from administering the estate.[7] This gives you time to take legal advice to see whether it is worth challenging the will on grounds of lack of testamentary capacity, lack of knowledge and approval or undue influence. Did the aged parent actually sign the new will or were they helped to sign it? Did he or she have mental capacity at the time? Was a medical report prepared at the time to say so?

If you are successful in challenging the will in court, quite a protracted and emotional (and sometimes expensive) process, and one which is not easy because the main witness is no longer with you, the earlier will, if there is one, is likely to be reinstated. At worst, criminal proceedings could be brought against a person who has exercised undue influence or even committed forgery.

Even if you were to lose your case, you could still claim that your parent had not made 'reasonable financial provision' for you and your siblings.[8] But all of this needs careful investigation and sound legal advice.

Keeping a will safe, but available

If a solicitor is nominated as an executor, they should hold the original signed will for safekeeping. You should keep a copy of your will in your death file (*see above*). Whether you keep the original yourself or a copy, it should be kept somewhere safe, but available. Some close member of your family needs to know where it is. Details of the solicitor should also be kept in writing.

You can also store your will with your bank or at the HM Courts and Tribunals (HMCTS) storage facility.[9]

Step 4: Make an Advance Decision (Living Will)

See example on p 297

What is an Advance Decision?

An Advance Decision is a written record of your wish to **refuse medical treatment** in the future, if and when you no longer have mental capacity to refuse treatment yourself.[10] It is a legally binding decision by you to refuse treatment.[11] That treatment will often include **life-sustaining treatment** (which could keep you alive).

To die will be an awfully big adventure.

J M Barrie, *Peter Pan* (1928)

It is different from (and more effective than) a Do Not Resuscitate notice (*see p 26*).

An Advance Decision is sometimes known informally as 'a living will'. It is also commonly known in England and Wales (where it is governed by statute: sections 24–26, Mental Capacity Act 2005) as an **Advance Decision to Refuse Treatment (ADRT)**.

There are different provisions in Scotland and Northern Ireland (*see p 28*).

An example of an Advance Decision (for England and Wales) is set out on *p 297*. It suggests:

- possible circumstances in which you might wish to refuse life-sustaining treatment (and receive palliative care instead)
- the sort of treatments, such as CPR, that you might wish to refuse, and
- reasons for expressing these wishes

It is a general principle of law and practice that people have a right to consent to or refuse medical treatment.[12] An Advance Decision is your opportunity to express your wishes to refuse specific treatment.

You do not have to make an Advance Decision; it is entirely up to you whether you do or not. If you decide not to, you will be leaving this kind of decision to be made in the future by healthcare professionals in your best interests. Or you can make a health and welfare Lasting Power of Attorney (a Welfare Power of Attorney in Scotland) so that those nominated by you will be able to make decisions on your behalf (*see pp 31–40*).

At the time of making an Advance Decision you must have the mental capacity (*see pp 43–51*) to make decisions.

The Advance Decision document will be used only when you are judged to be no longer able to make your own decisions about treatment or to communicate your wishes. It gives your carers and healthcare team clinical and legal instructions about your treatment choices, as if you were still able to make them.

You can only give instructions about *refusing* treatment. You cannot request in an Advance Decision that specific treatment be *provided*.[13]

You should discuss the document in advance (while you still have mental capacity) with close family and possibly your GP. If you discuss this with your GP, the GP can also consider your wishes for the future in the context of your treatment in the past. These are important decisions; you need to be properly informed of the implications.

The format for an Advance Decision

There is no special form for this. It may be expressed in 'laymen's terms'. But if it's to be applicable to life-sustaining treatment, the Advance Decision document must be:

- in writing
- signed and dated by you
- signed by a witness

An Advance Decision need not be in writing if it does not direct itself to life-sustaining treatment. For the purposes of this chapter, however, it is assumed that the maker of an Advance Decision is likely to have life-sustaining treatment in mind. Such a decision *must* be in writing.

The contents of an Advance Decision

It will be legally binding at the time of use and applicable, if:

- it is in the correct format (as above)
- you clearly had mental capacity at the time of making it
- you made it of your own free will, uninfluenced by anyone else
- you have not done anything since to suggest you have changed your mind
- you specified clearly which treatments you wish to refuse
- you explained the circumstances in which you wish to refuse them
- it clearly applies to the situation in hand
- it contains a statement that it applies even if your life is at risk

It would also be helpful to include in the Advance Decision document:

- your name and address
- your date of birth
- your next of kin or other close relative
- your GP's name, address and phone number
- your NHS number

and, last but not least,

- your reasons for making the specific decisions in the document (this adds weight to your intentions)

The circumstances of refusing treatment: the 'triggering event'

You may wish to refuse life-sustaining treatment in the event of:

- brain injury, including but not limited to stroke, vegetative or minimally conscious states
- diseases of the central nervous system (including but not limited to motor neurone disease, Parkinson's disease and Huntington's disease)
- dementia, including Alzheimer's disease
- any terminal illness

It is your decision which you choose. You don't have to choose any if you don't want to.

The treatment to be refused

There are many forms of life-sustaining treatment that you may choose to refuse, for example artificial ventilation (when you can't breathe on your own), clinically assisted nutrition and hydration (CANH) (being given food and drink by tube when you can't take them by mouth), antibiotics (to help fight off infection) or chemotherapy (cancer treatment).

Perhaps the most common decision people take is to refuse cardiopulmonary resuscitation (CPR).[14] **CPR** is treatment when you have stopped breathing (respiratory arrest) and/ or your heart has stopped beating (cardiac arrest). The latter is more common in later life. It is the most extreme form of medical emergency and requires immediate action.

CPR may involve one or more of the following:

- chest compressions
- blowing air or oxygen into the lungs (intubation)
- electrical shocks (defibrillation)

CPR often involves violent and repeated chest compressions (even to the frail and very elderly). It sometimes involves electrical shocks to stimulate the heart (defibrillation) and other forms of emergency treatment. Statistics on the survival rate in these circumstances vary. It is said by the NHS to be 20% or less, or less than 10% for out-of-hospital resuscitation attempts, and, of course, it reduces with age.[15] Even successful CPR can cause disabling complications such as fractured ribs (particularly with the elderly), damage to the liver or spleen or brain damage.

A risk to life

You *must* make it clear in writing that you are refusing the specified type of treatment *even if there is a risk to life.*

Treatment you cannot refuse

It is generally believed that an Advance Decision cannot refuse basic or essential care which is needed to keep a person comfortable and, in fact, the government Code of Practice says so.[16] This would include warmth, shelter, the offer of food and water by mouth, the control of distressing symptoms and washing and bathing. However, the relevant statute for England and Wales (the Mental Capacity Act 2005) does not specifically say so.

Unlawful wishes: euthanasia and assisted dying

An Advance Decision cannot be used to request that your life be ended. Euthanasia and assisted dying are illegal in the UK. They could lead to serious criminal charges. Suicide or attempted suicide is not a crime, but encouraging or assisting it is a crime. Keep an eye on this as a bill is about to go through parliament.[17]

Changing your mind: amend or withdraw your Advance Decision

Remember that while you have mental capacity you can change your mind at any time about any aspect of your Advance Decision. You can cancel or amend it if you wish to. To be on the safe side, any cancellation or changes should be written down, signed and witnessed.

In any event you may wish to review your choices from time to time.

A wrong decision isn't forever; it can always be reversed. The losses from a delayed decision are forever; they can never be retrieved.

J K Galbraith, *A Life in our Times* (1981)

Legally binding

If the Advance Decision is in proper form, it is legally binding. It *must* therefore be followed by carers and healthcare professionals even if they believe it is contrary to your 'best interests'. It is your choice. Your wishes must be complied with.

On the other hand, it should be noted that if you made the Advance Decision when you had mental capacity and also made a Lasting Power of Attorney (LPA) for health and care decisions when you had capacity, but have since lost capacity, it is likely that the LPA will prevail. The LPA will definitely prevail if made after the Advance Decision. This means that the 'attorney' under the LPA should *take into account your wishes* in the Advance Decision, but they do not, in the end, have to follow them. But it may depend upon the wording in the LPA. The relationship between an Advance Decision and an LPA is not straightforward. In an extreme position, expert legal advice may need to be obtained.

If there is a dispute about the Advance Decision, for example between doctors and family, a court may have to decide. The Court will decide whether the maker of the Advance Decision had mental capacity at the time the document was made, whether it is a valid document and whether it applies to the present medical situation.[18] The relevant courts are:

- the Court of Protection (England and Wales)
- the Sheriff Court (Scotland)
- the High Court (Northern Ireland)

Make the document readily available

In emergency circumstances, the Advance Decision document must be available at short notice. It should be kept with your GP and hospital medical records. A copy should be held by your next of kin and close family relatives as well as carers. For ease of reference a copy should be kept in your ON DEATH file (*see pp 10-11*).

In case of sudden emergency, of course, healthcare professionals may have no time to find out if there is a valid Advance Decision in existence and what it says. They need not delay emergency treatment in order to try and find out.

If you wish, you can carry a card on you, stating that you have made an Advance Decision.

Check life insurance policies

If you have life insurance policies you should check that they remain unaffected by an Advance Decision.

The difference between an Advance Decision and a Do Not Resuscitate notice (DNR)

Most people have heard of the term Do Not Resuscitate (or DNR).

A DNR notice used to be one way that a person could express their wishes in advance not to receive CPR (cardiopulmonary resuscitation) in time of emergency, usually cardiac arrest. The person would notify their doctor and the request would be added to their medical records. This record became more commonly known as a DNACPR notice (Do not attempt cardiopulmonary resuscitation).

But a DNACPR (or DNR) was (and still is, where it is sometimes used) not so much about the wishes of the person/patient. It is in essence a clinical decision by a doctor to make a recommendation that CPR would not be the right course of action in a future emergency. It can be created by a clinician with or without the consent of the person. If the person has expressed their wishes in this way, they should be taken into account, but they are not binding in law.

For this reason and a number of other reasons, the DNACPR (or DNR) approach, particularly for a person wishing to refuse treatment, is no longer regarded as best practice.

If you want to express your wishes about future treatment, about CPR or any other emergency treatment, you are therefore now advised to make an **Advance Decision to Refuse Treatment (ADRT)**, as above.[19] From your perspective (as opposed to the clinician's), the advantages for making an ADRT rather than a DNACPR are clear-cut:

- an ADRT is legally binding; a DNACPR is not, although it is persuasive
- an ADRT can be more comprehensive and can allow you to refuse *any* emergency treatment, if you so wish; a DNACPR is limited to one type of treatment, CPR

- an ADRT can also be written by yourself and does not necessarily have to require the input of a doctor (unless capacity is in issue)

It is, however, generally good practice to have a discussion with your GP or doctor in charge of your healthcare about your wishes. That will give you the opportunity to consider, and maybe plan, treatment options (or refusals) together. But that is up to you. For example, a discussion with your GP or healthcare doctor could lead to an agreed treatment plan for the future, using the helpful Recommended Summary Plan for Emergency Care and Treatment (ReSPECT) process, which is now widely used (although not everywhere).[20] This process creates personalised recommendations for your clinical care and treatment in a future emergency in which you are unable to make or express choices.

Some places still use stand-alone DNACPR forms and there are a range of different, sometimes inconsistent, forms and processes used in the healthcare community. But one thing is clear: from the person/patient's perspective, the simplest and clearest way to express *your* wishes about emergency treatment in the future is to write an Advance Decision (ADRT). This is now the recommended approach.

While you have mental capacity, you have the right to refuse any medical treatment, including CPR, in future time of emergency, and at a time when you will have lost capacity to decide for yourself, even if that refusal results in your death. Your wishes in an Advance Decision (ADRT) for future care and treatment must be respected.

Expressing your wishes for future treatment

1. Discuss your wishes with your doctor
2. Work with your doctor to agree a plan; use the ReSPECT process (if available)
3. Write an Advance Decision (ADRT)

Growing old is like being increasingly penalised for a crime you haven't committed.

Anthony Powell, *A Dance to the Music of Time*

The four countries of the UK

STEP 4 above applies to **England and Wales**. The provisions about Advance Decisions in the Mental Capacity Act 2005 do not apply to Scotland and Northern Ireland.

In **Scotland** an Advance Decision is known as an Advance Directive (or AD). Unlike England and Wales, an Advance Directive is not recognised in an Act of Parliament. There is therefore no statutory basis for making an Advance Directive binding in law. Nevertheless, it is widely recognised as being highly persuasive in setting out your wishes to refuse certain medical treatments (including CPR) and it is likely that the common law would follow the patient's wishes if clearly expressed.

At the very least, Scots law states that the present and past wishes and feelings of an adult with capacity shall be taken into account.[21] They will therefore be carefully considered, if not necessarily followed. An Advance Directive, therefore, is a good way of attempting to ensure that your wishes are respected by doctors in the future, were you to become incapable of expressing them at the time.[22]

An Advance Directive in Scotland should be in a similar format to an Advance Decision (in England and Wales). Preferably, it should be in writing, signed, dated and witnessed. But it does not have to be. You can just tell your doctor your wishes to refuse treatment and they can be recorded in your medical notes.

In **Northern Ireland**, this type of document is sometimes known as an Advance Directive, but is more commonly known as an Advance Decision to Refuse Treatment (ADRT). It has no statutory basis,[23] but is considered to be persuasive. Although not legally binding, it is expected that the common law would be likely to recognise an ADRT in Northern Ireland if clearly expressed.[24]

DNACPR forms (in various formats) have been used in **Scotland** and **Northern Ireland**, but their use is now discouraged in favour of Advance Decisions or Directives.[25]

Leave it to the medics

There is, of course, no obligation to discuss or express any wishes about resuscitation or any other form of emergency treatment. Even if healthcare professionals ask you about CPR at the time that it may be used (and you have capacity), you do not have express any preference. You can leave it up to them.

If you choose to make an **Advance Decision to Refuse Treatment (ADRT)**, it should be:

- Your decision and yours alone
- Discussed in advance with your GP and close family (if you wish)
- In proper form (*see p XX*), signed, dated and witnessed
- Made when you have mental capacity
- Clear in stating when it should apply
- Clear in stating what type(s) of treatment you refuse
- Clear in stating that it applies even when there is a risk to life
- Legal (not requesting euthanasia or assisted dying)
- Known to and understood by close family
- Kept readily available

It may be said that disease generally begins that equality which death completes.

Dr Johnson, *the Rambler* (1750–2)

Step 5: Make an Advance Statement

See example on p 297

An Advance Statement is different from an Advance Decision (above).[26] An Advance Decision is used to *refuse* medical treatments. An Advance Statement (in England and Wales) is a statement of **your wishes** for the future, including wishes for your care, for personal treatment, wishes to express your likes and dislikes, and wishes for your funeral. (For funeral planning, *see pp 40–41*). Unlike an Advance Decision, an Advance Statement is not binding in law; it is only persuasive.

If the time comes when you no longer have mental capacity or if you are unable to communicate your wishes, your Advance Statement will help others, such as your partner, family, carers and health professionals, to know what your wishes are.

An Advance Statement therefore has no legal standing. But it can persuasively set out your 'wishes and feelings'[27] at a time when you have the capacity to do so. It can be a helpful and important guide for those who care for you when you can no longer express clearly your wishes and preferences, your likes and dislikes.

An example of an Advance Statement is set out on *p 297*.

A similar document, with persuasive but not binding effect, can also be made in Scotland and Northern Ireland. The term Advance Statement in Scotland, however, has a special meaning. If you have a mental health condition, you can make an Advance Statement when you are well, expressing your views about treatment if you were to become unwell or have difficulty expressing your views.[28]

Format of an Advance Statement

Your future wishes can be told to a close family member in person, although it is better to write them down as well as discussing them with a family member. They can always be altered at any time, in writing or orally.

Your Advance Statement should be:

- in writing (but does not have to be – it could be a recorded video)
- clearly expressed
- signed and dated
- discussed with a family member (if you wish)
- made available to close family members (so that they can refer to it when necessary)
- also kept in your ON DEATH file

Contents of an Advance Statement

It is up to you how much you want to put in your Advance Statement. You should state your preferences, wishes and requests clearly.[29] They may include any of the following or more:

- where you would like to be cared for, eg at home (if possible)
- relevant information about your health
- how you normally do things, such as shower or bath
- what sort of food and drink you prefer
- what sort of music you prefer
- what you like to watch on TV
- what newspaper you like to read
- how you want your values or religious beliefs to be respected
- what sort of funeral you would like

Step 6: Lasting Powers of Attorney (LPAs)

What is a Lasting Power of Attorney (LPA)?

The paragraphs here apply to the law and practice in England and Wales. There are different laws and practice on this topic in Scotland and Northern Ireland (*see pp 39–40*).

A Lasting Power of Attorney (LPA) allows you (the 'donor') to choose one or more persons, known as 'attorneys', to make decisions for you later in life if and when you are unable to make decisions for yourself.

There are two separate LPAs:

- **a health and welfare LPA**
- **a property and financial affairs LPA**

An LPA makes it easier for those who are close to you, such as your children, to help you in later years when the decision-making process becomes more difficult.

Decisions include consent to medical treatment, refusal of medical treatment, where you live, arrangements for care and managing your financial affairs.

A Lasting Power of Attorney is a legally binding document. You must be 18 or over and have mental capacity (the ability to make decisions) at the time of making it.

There are special forms for LPAs which you must use (*see pp 34–35*).

A completed LPA must be registered with the Office of the Public Guardian (OPG).[30]

This process is overseen by the OPG which provides a detailed, helpful guide (LP12), *Make and register your lasting power of attorney*. See also information on the gov.uk website, *Lasting power of attorney, being in care and managing finances* and *Make, register or end a lasting power of attorney*.

Choosing an attorney or attorneys

An attorney must be chosen wisely. It can be anyone of your choosing, such as your partner, a close relative, close friend, or a solicitor or accountant. Normally, it will be your partner or closest relative (often a child), the one likely to be caring or looking out for you when you are no longer able to make decisions for yourself. It should be someone you know well and who knows you well, someone you can trust.

It should be not only someone you trust, but also someone who is good at making decisions and who you believe knows you well enough to make wise decisions on your behalf. For financial affairs, it should be someone with the necessary skills and abilities.

You can nominate more than one attorney. If more than one, you must decide whether they can make decisions in the future on your behalf either 'jointly' (they must be in agreement) or 'jointly and severally' (if there are two, either can decide alone or both can decide together in agreement). Some decisions could be requested to be made jointly, some other decisions jointly and severally. It is up to you what you specify in the LPA.

Before nominating someone, discuss it with them. It is a serious responsibility which both you and the attorney(s) should consider carefully. The choice of attorney must be made carefully and wisely. The wrong choice of attorney can bring problems. The number of court cases in the Court of Protection raising issues of misuse by attorneys for elderly (or vulnerable younger) persons has risen substantially.[31]

You can also name a replacement attorney in case the nominated one dies. This is optional.

The two types of Lasting Power of Attorney (LPA)

You can choose to make one type or both or neither. There is no legal requirement to make either. They are separate and different LPAs.

(1) Health and welfare LPA

Use this LPA to give your attorney(s) the power to make decisions about:

- medical care
- life sustaining treatment
- where you live
- everyday life, for example diet, washing, dressing
- help and support

The attorney can only make decisions for you *after* you lose the ability (mental capacity) to make decisions for yourself.

(2) Property and financial affairs LPA

Use this LPA to give your attorney(s) the power to make decisions about money and property for you, for example:

- managing a bank or building society account
- paying household and other bills
- collecting benefits or a pension
- selling your home
- managing savings and investments

The attorney can only make decisions for you *after* you lose the ability (mental capacity) to make decisions for yourself, *unless* the LPA expressly permits the attorney to make financial decisions *before* you lose capacity.

An attorney has no power to make decisions after your death.

The Lasting Power of Attorney was formerly known as an Enduring Power of Attorney[32] (the term still currently used in Northern Ireland).

Forms

An LPA can be made online or in paper form. It must be made on the right form[33]:

- Form LP1H for health and care decisions
- Form LP1F for financial decisions

Attempts to modernise and speed up the rather cumbersome application process by digitisation were introduced by the Powers of Attorney Act 2023.[34]

- For online applications see the gov.uk website.[35]
- Forms can be downloaded for paper use or you can complete one online (after you have created an account online).
- A paper form can be obtained from the Office of the Public Guardian (OPG). If you need help or advice contact the OPG at:

customerservices@publicguardian.gov.uk
phone 0300 456 0300
textphone 0115 934 2778
PO Box 16185
Birmingham
B2 2WH
See gov.uk, *Office of the Public Guardian*

The form must be signed and dated by the maker, the attorney(s) (including a replacement attorney, if there is one) and a witness.[36]

Certification

The form must also be signed by a further independent person, a 'certificate provider', who confirms that you make the LPA by choice and understand what you are doing. A certificate provider will be somebody you have known for at least two years, such as a friend, neighbour or colleague. Or a professional, such as your GP or solicitor.

These provisions are necessary in their detail, if perhaps a little complicated, because this is an important step to take.

Registration (and cost)

Once the form is completed and certified it must be provided to the Office of the Public Guardian for **registration**. For details on how to register an LPA see the gov.uk website. An LPA cannot be used until it is registered.

If a paper application has been made, the form should be sent for registration to:

The Office of the Public Guardian
PO Box 16185
Birmingham
B2 2WH

The **cost** for registration of each LPA is currently £82 (£164 for both LPAs).[37] LPAs are popular, so registration can take 'up to 16 weeks', according to the Government website,[38] although there have been reports of delays beyond that period, with the official time estimate having doubled in three years. Do not use a commercial website which claims that they can, for a larger fee, speed up your application for registration – they can't.

The Public Guardian may refuse to register an LPA if it is not in proper form, properly completed and certified, or if there is a valid notice of objection to it being registered. That objection might have to be considered by the Court of Protection. The Court also supervises alleged issues of misuse by attorneys.

Certified copies

Yet another step will help to guarantee that a copy of your LPA (not the original) is genuine. You can certify the bottom of each page of a copy (or more than one copy) with the words: *I certify this is a true and complete copy of the corresponding page of the original Lasting Power of Attorney.* Then sign and date every page. Or a solicitor or notary can certify the copy for you.

View an LPA online

Using paper documents and the post for verification of the authenticity of an LPA can sometimes be a cumbersome process. As an alternative, LPAs can be checked online using an **access code** supplied by the attorney or donor. This gives third party organisations, such as banks and utility companies, relatively easy access to an LPA in order to verify its authenticity (although some still require seeing a physical document).

First, the attorney or donor has to sign in to the Use an LPA Service to create an account: go to gov.uk, *Use a lasting power of attorney.*

Once the online account has been opened, the attorney and donor can:

- ask for an activation key (if not been given one or lost or expired)
- add an LPA

- view an LPA summary
- allow people or organisations to view an LPA
- keep track of those given access to an LPA

If the LPA was registered after 17 July 2020, the activation key should have been in the letter confirming that the LPA had been registered.

Only LPAs registered on or after 1 January 2016 can be 'viewed' online: see gov.uk, *Using the View an LPA Service* (May 2024). To view an LPA, a third-party organisation needs to obtain a 13-character-long 'LPA access code', provided by the attorney or donor.[39]

LPAs registered before 1 January 2016 are not available online. A paper version will have to be used to verify the LPA.

This online process applies only to LPAs registered in England and Wales.

Amendment and revocation

In legal terms an LPA is a deed, therefore it can only be revoked or amended by another deed.[40]

An LPA can be *amended* by the maker/donor (who still has capacity) in a written document known as a 'partial deed of revocation'.

An LPA can be *revoked* by the maker/donor (who still has capacity) by a formal 'deed of revocation'. It is automatically revoked on the death of the donor. An attorney has no authority from that point on.

Further details

For further information on all the technical aspects of LPAs, see Office of the Public Guardian, *Make and register your lasting power of attorney, a guide* (LP12); gov.uk, *Make, register or end a lasting power of attorney*; nhs.uk, *Lasting power of attorney*; ageuk.org.uk, *Power of attorney*; Mencap Trust Company, *Guides for lasting power of attorney*.

Making decisions

When the time comes and you no longer have the ability (mental capacity) to make decisions for yourself, your attorney will make decisions for you. An attorney must always act in your best interests.

If your elderly mother, for example, has executed a property and financial affairs LPA, she can still choose to make a gift to anyone she wants, so long as she has mental capacity to make the particular decision. The mere fact that a property and financial affairs LPA has been completed and registered cannot stop her from making her own choices however unwise they seem to you. If a 'gentleman' friend receives an expensive gift from her, there is very little you can do about it, if she has mental capacity for that particular decision. She is free to do what she likes with her own money. You could speak to her or speak to him with her permission, but a gift is a gift unless she lacks capacity or there is an element of fraud or undue influence. If there is fraud or undue influence, the police may help or action can be taken in the County Court to recover the 'gift'.

The attorney can act on her behalf usually only when she has lost mental capacity, although a property and financial affairs LPA may specify that the attorney can make certain decisions while she still has capacity. It will be assumed that she still has mental capacity until it is established otherwise, sometimes by medical evidence from her GP. In some instances it may become obvious that she really needs help making a decision. If at any time you suspect that she lacks mental capacity, you could seek medical advice to confirm it.

Once it is established that she lacks mental capacity, the nominated attorney can act on her behalf and make decisions, even important decisions, for her. When an attorney is about to make an important decision, the organisation in question, for example, a bank or hospital, will need to see a copy of the LPA. They may wish to see the original or a certified copy, or an 'access code' may be enough.

If you lose mental capacity (for example after a stroke), your partner or child has no legal authority to make decisions on your behalf unless there is an LPA in place, although in practice many day-to-day decisions have to be made. If there is no LPA in place, the Court of Protection may make the decision or appoint a 'deputy' to decide on your behalf. The Court's choice of that person will be made in your best interests. It could be a partner or close relative or close friend, sometimes a younger rather than older person, so that they will outlive you. Or it could be a professional person such as a solicitor.

The legal relationship between an Advance Decision and an LPA is discussed above (*see pp 20, 24-25*). This can be a difficult area. If in doubt, seek legal advice from a solicitor specialising in this field of law.

Separate laws for Scotland and Northern Ireland

The devolved countries of Scotland and Northern Ireland have their own laws on this topic.

Scotland – The procedure in Scotland is different. An LPA is called *a power of attorney*. Anyone can set up a continuing (financial) and/or welfare power of attorney nominating a specific person, the attorney, to make decisions for you in the future when you become incapable of making them yourself.[41]

There is no special form for use. Detailed guidance and a typical example of a power of attorney document are provided by the Office of the Public Guardian (Scotland) on their website. A completed power of attorney document must be registered with the Office of the Public Guardian (Scotland).

Guidance for attorneys is provided in the Scottish Government's Code of Practice for *Continuing and welfare attorneys* (2018). Scotland also has its own mental capacity provisions. They are set out in the Adults with Incapacity (Scotland) Act 2000.

Northern Ireland – Future provisions on lasting powers of attorney, including formalities similar to LPAs in England and Wales, such as forms and registration with the Public Guardian, are set out in the Mental Capacity Act (Northern Ireland) 2016. But these provisions have not yet been brought into force.

Meanwhile, enduring powers of attorney continue to be used. See the Northern Ireland Government website at nidirect.gov.uk, *Managing your affairs and enduring power of attorney*.

An enduring power of attorney (EPA) enables you to choose a person or persons (attorney(s)) to deal with your property and affairs in the event that you lose capacity to make decisions for yourself.

It should be noted that an EPA is limited to property and affairs. It does not include your health and welfare.

An EPA must be in the prescribed form.[42] It must be registered with the High Court (Office of Care and Protection), but only when the attorney believes you are becoming incapable of managing your affairs.[43] At this point it *endures*, after you lack capacity.

Step 7: Plan for Inheritance Tax

If you are fortunate enough to have substantial assets to leave in your will, you should consider planning for inheritance tax (**see pp 138–140**).

Step 8: Plan for Your Funeral

Expressing your wishes

If you wish to, and only if you wish to, you can make plans for your own funeral. The expression 'It's your funeral' finally has some meaning. You should tell your close family what you would like.

You can either:

- write it down as part of your will or Advance Statement (if you choose to make one) (**see above**)
- write it down separately, or
- just tell your close family orally

It is better to write down your wishes in case they get forgotten. None of this is legally binding (except in your will), but your wishes should at the very least be considered, if not followed. For your family, it is not always easy to talk about these things. But if you, as the older family member, are willing to talk about it, it helps everybody to know your wishes. Or at least they can be found after death, written down in your ON DEATH file.

What sort of wishes?

You do not have to plan or discuss every detail. It is entirely your choice whether you do or do not. But you might like to express your wishes on any of the following:

- burial or cremation
- what kind of service or event
- religious requirements (if any)
- where it will be held
- who will be invited
- hymns or songs, music, readings, speeches etc.
- what sort of 'wake'

I remember the broad smiles on the faces of mourners as we left a funeral service in a village hall to the rousing chant of the Leeds United anthem, my late friend's particular wish. He would have been smiling too.

At another, tea was the only drink provided at the wake. Those who wanted to toast the memory of our friend sloped off after a while to the nearby pub. Everybody was catered for.

Step 9: Write a Short History

Leave behind a memoir. Write a short history of your life and family. However brief it is, write down something about:

- your parents, grandparents, other relatives (including full names and dates)
- your early, middle and later life
- your work and leisure, your interests and pursuits
- some memorable dates
- your beliefs and credo (if you wish)

This short history of your life and family is for the benefit of your family and heirs. And it doesn't have to be so short – it's up to you. My parents gave me a couple of sheets of paper each about their past and family before they died. I wish now that I had asked for more. I have spent much time trying to fill out their histories with rather more detail. I am working on my own, too. A little family history is a good thing. It also gives a feeling for you of looking back, hopefully with satisfaction, over what is done and dusted but not forgotten.

Ideas for your short history

- Dates
- People/names
- Places/homes
- Events
- Education
- Work
- Stories
- Photos
- Documents
- Favourites (books, music etc)

If you want to do a proper job and create your own autobiography, there are websites which, for a fee, will help you.[44] You could also create a video, or a 'virtual memorial', even an AI chatbot (known as a griefbot or deathbot) that will mimic you and 'tell your story after you've gone'.

All men [and women], *whatever be their condition… should write the tale of their life with their own hand.*

Benvenuto Cellini[45]

Mental Capacity

In every one of the steps above, the issue of mental capacity is extremely important. You must have mental capacity before you can make:

- a will
- an Advance Decision
- an Advance Statement
- a Lasting Power of Attorney

In fact you must have mental capacity for any significant decision you make. Without it, your decision may not stand. It could, for example, be ignored by others such as healthcare professionals. But if you clearly have mental capacity, all decisions, whether on everyday matters or something more important, are yours to make and should not be countermanded.

This is the position in England and Wales. For Northern Ireland and Scotland, *see below pp 48–49*.

Rule your mind or it will rule you.

Horace, *Carmina* (c. 20 BC)

What is *mental capacity*?[46]

Mental capacity is the **ability to make decisions for yourself**. It is also the ability to consent to acts of care or treatment. In law, it is *assumed* that you have mental capacity unless established otherwise.[47] These and other principles of mental capacity are defined for England and Wales in the Mental Capacity Act 2005 and discussed in the Mental Capacity Act Code of Practice. It is all about the capacity to make decisions, whether everyday or more significant.[48]

As the Code states, a person's capacity (or lack of capacity) refers specifically to their capacity to make a particular decision at the time it needs to be made.

Causes of mental incapacity

You lack capacity if you are **unable to make a decision** for yourself because of a **temporary or permanent impairment or disturbance** in the functioning of the mind or brain. This may result from dementia, for example, or from a stroke or from brain damage, from a mental health problem or from a disability.

For the purposes of this book, mental capacity is considered in the context of older persons. But the principles of mental capacity (or the lack of it) apply to all persons aged 16 or over.

Test for mental incapacity

The law says that you are **unable to make a decision at the time** if *any one or more* of the following four tests applies.

1 You are unable to understand the information relevant to the decision
2 You are unable to retain that information
3 You are unable to use or weigh that information as part of the decision-making process, or
4 You are unable to communicate your decision

Equally, if you are unable to make a particular decision, the cause (for testing mental incapacity) must be impairment or disturbance in the functioning of the mind or brain.

It is important to note that you are still capable of making a decision if you are able to retain the information only for a short period. Also, if you make an unwise decision that does not make you incapable. And it will not be decided that you lack capacity unless all practical steps have first been taken to support you.

It is also important to note that a person may be able to make decisions at some times but not at others. A person with a mental health problem may be capable of making decisions when well, but not when unwell. Or a person may be able to make some decisions but not others. For example, a person may be capable of making everyday decisions about what clothes to wear, but not more important decisions about finances.

For these reasons, the test of mental capacity, whether you have it or not, must be made for each decision at the time in question.

Consequence of mental incapacity

When you are judged not to have mental capacity, others may make decisions for you. These include close family, social carers and healthcare professionals. It also includes a person acting under a Lasting Power of Attorney.

A decision made on your behalf when you lack mental capacity, must be made *in your best interests*. This applies to anyone making the decision.

In making the decision in your best interests, any wishes you expressed in the past should be taken into account, especially if you have made an Advance Decision to refuse medical treatment (ADRT) or an Advance Statement. If a valid Advance Decision is in place, it must be followed; there is no best-interests decision to be made.

Decisions by others *in your best interests* may include:

- everyday decisions eg clothing, food, hygiene, mobility
- healthcare and treatment decisions (including refusal of life-sustaining treatment)
- where to live
- financial decisions eg banking, gifts, purchases, household services and utilities

Who judges?

In practice, the assessment of capacity or lack of it is made by **the person most suitable**. On a daily basis a carer may make everyday decisions, for example about meals or clothing. On more significant decisions your GP or hospital doctor will make the assessment of capacity. Sometimes other healthcare professionals may make the assessment, for example a psychiatrist who is a specialist in old age. A district nurse may make the assessment when medical decisions need to be made. At hospital, having to make an important decision may lead to an assessment on capacity by a multi-disciplinary team. Or a social care team may make a significant care decision.

A solicitor may make decisions about legal transactions, such as making a will (*see above*), after taking account of circumstances and the views of close family, and often assisted by medical advice.

In all these cases the more information made available for the assessor (and related to the decision in question) the better. This includes consideration of all relevant circumstances and the wishes (if any) expressed by the person when having capacity. It is important to consult others.

There may well be obvious features of the person's life which indicate a clear mental capacity to make decisions. For example, if they are still in work or a voluntary occupation. Or if that person cares for an elderly relative, partner or grandchild or has other regular aspects of their life which show clear capacity. Mental incapacity should never be assumed; quite the reverse. It must always be assumed that the person has mental capacity unless established otherwise.

If there is a dispute or uncertainty as to whether a person lacks mental capacity, ultimately the Court of Protection (in England and Wales) will decide. The Court may appoint a Deputy to make the more important decisions for a person who lacks mental capacity, but only if the Court is unable to make the decision in question itself.

A Deputy is a person who is reliable and trustworthy and has the appropriate skills for the particular decision or decisions. The appointed Deputy could be a family member or someone who knows the person well. Or the Deputy could be an independent person or an expert in the particular field. It could be the local authority's Director of Adult Services. There is a panel of professionals, mostly solicitors, who specialise in this area of law, which the Court can draw upon. A Deputy must act in the best interests of the person. See Chapter 8 of the Mental Capacity Act Code of Practice.

Assessing mental capacity (or the lack of it) for a particular decision

1. What is the nature of the decision to be made?
2. Can the person be supported in making that decision?
3. Is the person capable of making the decision in question?
4. If incapable, is it because of an impairment or disturbance in the functioning of the mind or brain?
5. Who is best placed to assess capacity for this particular decision?
6. Is a professional assessment required?
7. If capacity is assessed as lacking, action on the decision must be made in the best interests of the person

Decisions made by others: the *best interests* test

If you are assessed to lack mental capacity, all decisions must be made on your behalf by the appropriate person or team *in your best interests*. This includes taking into account your views expressed before you lost capacity and all circumstances which you would have taken into account if you had been making the decision yourself with the necessary capacity. If possible, others should be consulted too.

The best interests test does not apply if you have made an Advance Decision to refuse certain medical treatment (*see pp 19-29*). Your wishes in an Advance Decision (in England and Wales) must be respected even if the medical experts consider they are not in your best interests. Your wishes cannot be overridden.

For the law in Northern Ireland and Scotland, *see below*.

What is in your best interests is not a static concept. Your best interests may change over time. They should therefore be reviewed from time to time. Records should be kept of important decisions, particularly by professionals. The record should state the reasons for the best-interests decision and the factors taken into account.

If there is a disagreement about what is at any particular time in the best interests of the person who has lost mental capacity – for example, a difference of family views – the decision-maker will have to find a way of balancing these views or deciding between them. Ultimately, if necessary, the Court of Protection (in England and Wales) will decide.

If there is no one available to discuss a major decision about medical treatment or long-term residential placements, an Independent Mental Health Advocate (IMCA) should be consulted. In England and Wales IMCAs are appointed through local authorities in conjunction with the NHS. There are different arrangements in Northern Ireland.

Key points to remember

Remember that one of the key principles of the Mental Capacity Act 2005 (in England and Wales) is that you are **assumed to have mental capacity** unless and until it is proved otherwise. In legal terms, the test is whether it is reasonably believed that you lack capacity.[49]

And it must also be remembered that assessing capacity (or the lack of it) is specific to the **particular decision** and the time when it is to be made.[50]

Northern Ireland and Scotland[51]

Similar statutory principles would apply in **Northern Ireland** but have not yet been brought into force: they are set out in the Mental Capacity Act (Northern Ireland) 2016, much of which is based upon the Mental Capacity Act 2005, which applies in

England and Wales. The law on lack of capacity is therefore based mainly on the common law principles. These are, in any event, not dissimilar to the Act. In relation to your care and treatment, action may only be taken in your best interests when there is a reasonable belief that you lack capacity to consent to what is proposed. In case of dispute, the High Court will decide.

In Northern Ireland, under the common law, a person is presumed to have capacity unless 'some impairment or disturbance of mental functioning renders the person unable to make a decision whether to consent or to refuse treatment'.[52] The best interests test applies.

In **Scotland**, mental capacity is defined differently. In broad terms, the Adults with Incapacity (Scotland) Act 2000 requires two questions to be answered: (1) Is the person incapable of making, communicating, understanding or retaining the memory of decisions? And (2), if so, is that because of mental disorder or of inability to communicate because of physical disability?[53] In a case where capacity is disputed, the Sheriff Court can decide. An intervention in the affairs of an adult can be made only if it will 'benefit the adult'.[54]

Deprivation of Liberty Safeguards (DoLS)

A footnote on mental capacity (in England and Wales only): in summary, if a person in a care home or hospital lacks capacity (as outlined above), their local authority can authorise (without having to go to court) that they be deprived of their liberty and restrained. The deprivation of their liberty must be necessary in order to keep them safe from harm.

These authorisations by the local authority are known as Deprivation of Liberty Safeguards, or DoLS for short.

Typical examples include bars on the windows to prevent elderly dementia patients from exiting a care home or internal locks on the doors to stop people walking alone into the street. In one case, a distressed care-home resident with dementia said he was going home, not remembering that he had sold his flat when he moved into the care home. He was found agitated and lost, wandering along a nearby main road.

This is a complicated (and important) subject. I shall do no more than summarise some of the key points. Article 5 of the European Convention on Human Rights (*see pp 258-259*) protects everyone's 'right to liberty ... save ... in accordance with a procedure prescribed by law'. The statute law on DoLS prescribes an exception to that right: Schedules A1, AA1 and 1A of the Mental Capacity Act 2005 (as inserted by the Mental Health Act 2007).

Care homes and hospitals can apply to their local authority for a DoLS authorisation when they are concerned about the safety of a resident or patient.

The local authority will then make an assessment, which should involve consulting the person's family, friends and carers. Before an authorisation is given, attempts should be made to see if the restraint needed could be achieved in some other way, 'a way that is less restrictive of the person's rights and freedom of action'.[55] An authorisation can be given only if it is in the 'best interests' of the person. It must be necessary and proportionate. 'All the relevant circumstances' have to be considered.[56] These include how a person lives and is cared for, the current circumstances, as well as past and present wishes and feelings, and including any Advance Decision (*see above*).[57]

If the local authority gives an authorisation, the care home or hospital is permitted to restrain the person in their own interests. Without the authorisation, restraint would be unlawful and could amount to false imprisonment, assault or trespass to the person. An authorisation can be challenged in the Court of Protection.

DoLS do not apply to persons living in their own home in the community (including supported accommodation). They cannot be the subject of deprivation of liberty, except by order of the Court of Protection. In 2022 there were over 6,000 applications in England and Wales to the Court of Protection for deprivation of liberty orders. By contrast, in England alone, in the years 2022-23 there were over 300,000 applications for DoLS. 56% of these were not granted, mostly because of the person's change of circumstances, such as being discharged from a short-term stay in hospital.[58]

In 2019 an Act of Parliament introduced Liberty Protection Safeguards (LPS) as a future replacement for DoLS.[59] However, the implementation of LPS has been delayed indefinitely. It is not known if or when LPS will replace DoLS.

How best to proceed if you do have mental capacity

It is therefore very important to make decisions for the future at a time when you do have mental capacity. Hopefully you will never lose it, but it is always a possibility. You might at some later date have a disabling stroke or gradually develop dementia. Now is the time, therefore, to take steps and prepare in advance. Consider these **NINE STEPS** when you are younger and hopefully fitter. Take time to consider what you feel your wishes are.

Keeping up the appearance of having all your marbles is hard work, but important.

Sara Gruen, *Water for Elephants*[60]

Top Ten Tips: For Expressing Your Wishes for the Future and Making Your Voice Heard

1	**Plan for the future now (while you have mental capacity, in case you lose it).** It is important that your wishes should be heard later in life at a time when you may lose mental capacity (eg because of a stroke, heart attack or developing dementia).
2	**Think about your wishes and discuss them with those close to you.** Consider the medical and social options and make choices so that you are empowered, and let your close family know what your wishes are.
3	**Consider how you want your finances managed in your lifetime.** Discuss it with a trusted relative or friend and set something down in writing.
4	**Making a will** is essential to express your wishes as to whom shall inherit
5	**Consider making an Advance Decision to Refuse Treatment (ADRT)**, a living will, to express your wishes (if you lose mental capacity) to refuse treatment in a medical emergency
6	**Consider making a Lasting Power of Attorney (LPA)** to allow someone close to you, whom you can trust, to manage: • your health and welfare, and/or • your property and financial affairs
7	**Consider making an Advance Statement** to express your wishes for the future about care and personal treatment
8	**Plan for your funeral** (if you want to)
9	**Write a short history** about yourself and your family
10	**Create an ON DEATH file** for key documents and other important information. Keep it in a safe place.

CHAPTER 2

Money

Money lays waste to cities; it sets men to roaming from home; it seduces and corrupts honest men and turns virtue to baseness; it teaches villainy and impropriety.

Sophocles, *Antigone* (c.340 BC)

Let's not be quite so pessimistic. Money is not everything – 'Money can't buy you love' – but we all need it. So a little bit of organisation and management, as well as understanding and checking your proper entitlement, can sometimes help provide extra comfort and peace of mind for older persons. We can definitely be more positive than Sophocles.

The purpose of this chapter is to look at ways of managing and handling money in as simple a manner as possible, and to the best effect. It also looks at solving money problems. A list of ten top tips is set out at the end of the chapter.

This may be a good time for making the best of your money. The incomes of pensioners used to be rising at a rate faster than those of the working-age population, with incomes slightly higher than non-pensioners. Not anymore. According to the Institute for Fiscal Studies, the 30-year 'onward march of pensioners' seems to have halted and the upward trend stopped some years ago: 'Perhaps we have finally reached peak pensioner.'[1] More care and thought may therefore need to be given to looking after your finances.

This is not financial advice about where to put your money or how to invest it. Only a qualified financial adviser can do that, one who is formally approved by the Financial Conduct Authority (FCA). It is more about tips for sensible financial organisation, tips for dealing well with what you have, however much or little that may be (and particularly in times of higher inflation and higher energy prices).

One tip which is often given is that you should only take advice on what to do with your money if you can **trust** that person absolutely. That may be a close family member or trusted friend or an independent financial adviser (IFA) who has been recommended to you and upon whom you are sure you can rely. Good financial advice can be invaluable. It can put your mind at rest about the financial security of your future.

Start by getting organised.

When money is not a servant, it is a master.

Japanese proverb

Organise and Plan

Organise your files

Let us begin at the beginning. First, and this may sound obvious to some of you, make sure your files and documents are in order. Some of you may be completely organised digitally, with all necessary information and documentation stacked away on your computer, and good backup. But many people of my age, in their seventies and older, still rely very much on paperwork (when available): paper bills, utility bills, pension statements, bank statements, invoices, insurance policies, etc. You will not be alone. It is said that less than one third of all financial services customers have actually gone paperless, despite the rise in online banking. There is still demand for paper records and resistance to digital records. People still seem to want something physical, easily accessible and harder to ignore. Perhaps they also wish to escape endless online registration and re-registration and avoid lost passwords and other login details.

It is very easy as you get older to leave documents lying around in piles – a lot of people do. But if you are trying to keep track of your money and bills, or a close relative is doing it for you or just helping you from time to time, it saves hours of work if you have your documents in order, properly filed and organised.

Most of the companies who send you this paper will want you to go paperless. It is cheaper for them for all your documents to be online (and, in green terms, saves on paper). But if you are more comfortable with paper, as many older people are, ensure as much as possible that you keep receiving all the necessary paperwork through the post. And if you do that, you should make sure that you file everything in easily accessible files. It is a small task, if done once a week or once a month. And it makes looking after your money much easier. If you are worried about an unusually high electricity bill, well-organised paperwork means you can go back through recent bills and check much more easily.

And, to be frank, it is a lot easier for your family after your death, if you have left everything neatly organised and in one accessible place, if necessary labelled or colour-coded, with the latest document on top.

Organise your money

If you are fortunate enough to have acquired money for your later years, you may be happy having your money in all sorts of different banks and funds. To some extent there is, no doubt, wisdom in the old adage, 'Don't keep all your eggs in one basket.'

It is up to you whether you leave it like that or involve yourself in a little re-organisation. Many bank and building society accounts lie dormant, earning little or no interest. Some are untouched for many years and sometimes their owners just cannot be traced. There are so many of these that the government announced in 2018 that if accounts have not been touched for 15 years and the holders cannot be traced, the money will be given away to help homeless people and other causes. It was said that on average there was less than £100 in each account, but that over a four-year period £330 million would be available for charities, under the Dormant Assets Scheme.[2] There is a free online service for tracing lost accounts and savings: mylostaccount.org.uk. You will not lose your money from dormant accounts as long as you claim it.

One way of organising is to rationalise your accounts, maybe closing some and holding on to others, or opening others which earn more interest. For example, you may have opened an account with an attractive first-year offer of high interest. But after a year that rate will drop significantly. Leaving your money in that account after the first year will earn you very little.

An independent adviser could help you make the most of your money (*see pp 62–64*). After all, you may need sufficient funds for proper care in later life, as discussed in chapter 8.

Also remember that if you have funds in a bank account, the Financial Services Compensation Scheme protects that money only up to £85,000 per person per bank or building society, or £170,000 for a joint account.

Another way is to bring funds and pensions under one roof with an independent managed platform (sometimes called a wrap service).[3] You can manage your own funds, or part of them, and make your own investments, or, as most do, you can rely on professionals to do this for you. If you rely on a financial adviser to invest for you, the adviser can make investment changes with the platform's combined administration. This form of service manages the administration of your investments in one portfolio (or platform). It uses smart technology so that it is easier for you to keep an eye on your savings and investments. There are a number of platforms. You should take advice.

But it is entirely your choice, with or without help from others who you can trust, how you manage your money.

It is not advisable to play the stock market on your own unless you know what you are doing. And don't let anyone do it for you unless they are qualified to give advice. Don't invest in some attractive-sounding investment scheme unless you know precisely what it is all about and that it is absolutely genuine. If it sounds too good to be true (with a high rate of interest promised), it probably is. Never invest following a cold call over the phone. You need more than that, much more than that, to be sure that the investment opportunity is sound. If in doubt, don't. Better to be safe than sorry, as discussed in chapter 5.

Write a financial summary file

If you have the time, make a list of your money files. For example, make a list of the bank accounts which are active (not closed), with a summary of their contents. And then date the summary. It is good to be aware of your funds, particularly your income (and expenditure). That helps you to review and change them, if and when you wish. It will also be helpful to others on your death. If somebody is looking after your affairs, they should do the same. Even if your income is limited, a summary will always help.

And make sure that those you trust, and only those you trust, know where the summary and details are.

I keep my financial summary file in another file which is charmingly labelled *On Death* (*see p 10-11*). It contains a number of key documents and information for those who will be left behind when I die. The key documents and information listed there include:

- Will
- Key names and contact details: eg GP (with NHS card), probate solicitor
- Any Advance Decision, Advance Statement
- Any registered Lasting Power of Attorney
- Financial summary
- Family details, including birth/marriage certificates; brief family history

Contents of a Financial Summary File:

1. National insurance number (also used for State Pension reference)
2. Tax reference number
3. Accountant details (if you have one)
4. Independent Financial Adviser details (if you have one)
5. List of income, including
   - State Pension
   - Workplace pension(s)
   - Personal pension(s)
   - Benefits
   - Employment
   - Shares
   - Savings
   - Other
6. Bank/building society account(s) details
7. Insurance policies
8. Property (owned/rented) details

Devise a budget plan

Some people like to document their income and expenditure on a spreadsheet (or some other document), so that they can budget and plan for the present and the future, keeping control of their money. This is usually done on a monthly or annual basis, setting income against regular outgoings. The following is a fairly standard list of income and outgoings to measure the balance. It should help you to assess, for example, whether you are spending too much on a particular item and whether there are savings to be made.

Many of the outgoings are regular payments which can be assessed from bills as monthly sums. As you can see, it can all add up quite quickly. A budget plan will allow you to see whether any of your spending is necessary or wasteful, or whether you have scope to spend a little more.

A budget plan may put a check upon paying out for holidays that are too luxurious, restaurants you can't really afford, unaffordable hobbies, the accumulation of credit card debt, an over-ambitious mortgage or very expensive items of clothing. Do not hide your head in the sand if debt is mounting up. It is better to be on top of things than let them slide away. Take control.

On the other hand, if your budget chart shows that you can spend a little more, why not? There are also some apps that will work out income and expenditure for you.[4]

Some people budget using the 50:30:20 expenditure proportion ratio[5]:

- 50% for 'needs' (the essentials of everyday living)
- 30% for 'wants' (nights out, leisure etc)
- 20% for saving

Budget Plan

A. Income	Monthly/annual net £s
1 Pension(s)	
2 Work	
3 Savings	
4 Other	
Total	

B. Expenditure

		£s
(1) ESSENTIALS		
	(a) House, flat	
1	Mortgage/rent	
2	Council tax	
3	House/contents insurance	
4	Gas, electricity	
5	Water, sewage	
6	Broadband, TV, phone	
	Total	
	(b) Groceries	
7	Essential food, drinks, household goods	
	(c) Car	
8	Petrol, diesel, electric	
9	Insurance, VEL, MOT	
	Total	
(2) NON-ESSENTIALS		
10	Leisure, entertainment	
11	Hobbies, birthdays, Christmas etc	
12	Other	
	Total	
(3) SAVING FOR RAINY DAYS		
13	House repairs, decoration, new boiler	
14	Holiday	
15	Other	
	Total	
	TOTAL INCOME	
	TOTAL EXPENDITURE	
	BALANCE	

Taking Advice

*Advice is like mushrooms.
The wrong kind can prove fatal.*

EC McKenzie

An independent financial adviser (IFA)

If you have funds and you need to reorganise your money or help an older person to do so or if you need pension, investment or tax advice, you may need an independent financial adviser (IFA). You may do, you may not. If you are good at money you can be your own DIY money enthusiast. But if in doubt, take independent advice from a regulated adviser.

In a survey carried out by the *Financial Times*, 69% of their readers paid for financial advice whereas 31% did not. Of those who did not, many did not know where to find an adviser they could trust and many were put off by the cost. Quite a few liked to manage their own funds. Nearly half of those who found an adviser did so through the recommendation of a friend or family member and 79% were satisfied or very satisfied with the service they received. Surprisingly, more than half had changed their adviser.[6]

Which adviser?

Deciding which independent financial adviser to consult can be difficult. Plucking one from the internet may not be the best route. It may be wise to ask around. Ask a friend, preferably a trusted friend, or trusted relative who has an adviser they can recommend.

If necessary, have a 'beauty parade' until you find who suits you best. That means asking a small number of recommended financial advisers to visit you (or you can visit them, in person or online) and pitch their wares. This can be quite a personal thing, not just a financial decision, who you feel comfortable working with. Work out in advance what you want from an adviser. What you need is an adviser you can trust, an adviser you can work with, an adviser who understands your needs and tailors advice to those needs. Take your time and consider who suits you best.

You can search for a regulated financial adviser through independent websites such as:

- The Society of Later Life Advisers (SOLLA)
- unbiased.co.uk
- vouchedfor.co.uk

or through other websites which will list advisers local to you, such as:

- The Chartered Institute for Securities & Investments Wayfinder Tool
- Your Money

The government-supported website MoneyHelper is independent. It gives general advice on *Choosing a financial adviser*[7] and hosts a directory of regulated advisers, in particular retirement advisers. As they point out, not all financial advisers will be called IFAs. They may be called a pensions adviser, mortgage adviser, investment adviser or financial planner. But they should all be regulated by the Financial Conduct Authority (FCA): check the Financial Services Register on www.register.fca.org.uk.

Check with any adviser to see that they are strictly independent and that they are properly authorised (regulated by the FCA) to give the advice you seek.

What advice?

You will probably want face-to-face advice at first and annually (despite the rise of 'robo advice' services, which use artificial intelligence to assess your needs). In between meetings you should be satisfied by emails and online portfolio scrutiny.

You may need one-off advice or ongoing advice. Advisers fall into one of two categories: restricted or independent. Restricted advisers are, as the word suggests, limited to recommending only certain types of products including their own. Independent advisers (IFAs) have no such restraints. You may want pensions advice, investments advice, tax planning (particularly inheritance tax planning) or general portfolio advice.

Fees

Good financial advice must be paid for; there is no such thing as free independent advice. The most common complaint about financial advisers is a lack of transparency about fees. But in the right case it could well be worth paying for, and some advisers may give you a free introductory session. Make it clear to an adviser that you want to know from the start about fees: what you will be paying, what you will get for it and how much you must expect to be paying in the future. You may choose to pay expressly for the advice rather than have the money taken by the adviser from various transactions carried out on your behalf or a percentage of your assets (which could be very expensive). These are choices for you.

Plan for the future

You may wish to sit down with your financial adviser and plan for the future. Think about how best to organise your finances. This is something that can be done gradually, step by step. Remember that we now retire later in life and live longer. That requires more planning, more thinking about the future.

Address weaknesses in your finances and plan gradually to improve them. Make a list of what needs to be done in order of importance. For example:

- Have you put your bank statements and household bills in accessible order?
- Have you put money from low-income accounts into something that produces interest?
- Do you have sufficient life insurance?
- Have you considered inheritance-tax planning?

- Are there good financial reasons why you should consider marrying your partner? (*see pp 92–95*)
- Is there a property and financial affairs Lasting Power of Attorney in place?
- Could you get part-time work if you looked for it (and wanted it)?
- Have you worked on paying off loans or reducing credit card debts?

By being organised you should be able to reduce your worries and enjoy life more.

Income

Pensions and Benefits

For most people, pensions are the major if not the sole source of income in older age, whether the State Pension (currently from age 66), workplace pensions or personal pensions. It is important to get the best and make the best out of them. This is dealt with in much more detail in chapter 3.

Work and pray, live on hay,
You'll get pie in the sky when you die.

Joe Hill, *Preacher and the Slave* (song, 1911)

Work

For those past the State pensionable age (currently 66 years) there may be options for full- or part-time working, whether employed or self-employed. While many of pensionable age seek rewards other than financial ones, choosing to volunteer for charities and other organisations or help out in caring for grandchildren, partners or elderly relatives, others choose to or have to seek employment.

More older people are working. For the over-65s, the employment rate has doubled over the last 25 years. Nearly 1.5 million are in employment (mostly self-employed and part-time). That figure is nearly 500,000 for those aged 70 and over, and 53,000 for the over-80s.[8] The over-60s account for nearly a quarter of all adults who are self-employed.[9]

In addition to reducing your job from full-time to part-time or taking up freelance work or consulting in your field of expertise, *Rest Less*, a website for those over 50 looking for jobs, volunteer work or later life careers' advice and courses, suggests part-time jobs in some of the following areas are popular[10]:

Top part-time jobs:

1. Tutoring/education
2. Driving
3. Childcare
4. Hair and beauty
5. Admin
6. Retail

With the State Pension age going to rise in due course, with life expectancy increasing and with fewer 'gold-plated' workplace pensions, there will be more older people in the workforce than ever before. This growing workforce should be recognised, not only for its commercial potential – cruises, equity release, insurance, mobility aids, lotions and potions – but also for its contribution to the economy and society.

Whether work is undertaken through choice or not, the benefits of later life working include having more income, staying active, staying socially connected, having greater confidence and self-respect, and having a sense of fulfilment.

Savings and Investments

Where you put your savings and how you invest your money is a matter for you (and your financial adviser (IFA), if you have one). It is not my role in this book to advise you on investments, if you are fortunate enough to be able to afford them, whether they be stocks and shares, bonds, funds, property, bank or savings accounts, or something rather more unusual like art, wine or start-up tech companies. Unless you know your way around investments, you need expert independent financial advice for all of these options.

A few warnings:

- Act carefully if you do not take independent financial advice
- Look out for hidden charges; check fees
- Consider whether any income from investments may affect your tax band
- Remember that market investments, such as stocks and shares ISAs, can go down as well as up
- The greater the risk in an investment, the greater the potential return, but also the greater the potential loss
- Avoid investments that are too good to be true
- Don't act on investment 'advice' from a cold caller (*see pp 148-149*)
- Don't open emails about investments from 'companies' you have had no dealings with

A penny saved is a penny earned

English proverb

Avoid big risks?

It is often said that older people should avoid taking big, and some might say foolish, risks which may end disastrously. Researchers[11] have concluded that losing three quarters or more of your wealth within two years increases your risk of dying earlier by 50%, a risk described as being 'similar to the increase associated with a new diagnosis of coronary heart disease'.[12] 'It is an iron law of investment that risks are correlated with returns.'[13]

Financial balance may be better. Do not put all your eggs in one basket is often sound advice. And never take a cold call from anyone offering an investment or pension advice. Avoid highly 'attractive' returns, high percentage yields. Some are scams. Some are just hopeless promises. I talk about these in more depth in chapter 5.

ISAs

You may, however, wish to think about obvious saving vehicles such as ISAs, which provide tax-free income. You might, for example, like to start a little saving for a grandchild, using a Junior ISA (although note that a Junior ISA can be opened only by a parent or guardian).

ISAs, formerly known as PEPs, have been around for nearly 25 years. They are Individual Savings Accounts. Although ISAs have the advantage of being tax free on any interest/profits earned, they will be subject to inheritance tax (IHT). An ISA can be passed on to your spouse or civil partner tax-free, but not further, for example not to children.

The amount you can invest in an ISA each year is capped by the government. It is called the ISA allowance.

The current annual ISA allowance[14]

Cash ISA or Investment ISA – £20,000

Lifetime ISA – £4,000

Junior ISA – £9,000

Maximum annual limit – £20,000

You can put up to a total of £20,000 each year into one or more ISAs (although not different types of ISA). Many people pay regularly, mostly monthly, as a relatively pain-free way of saving. Although annual contributions are capped, there is no total maximum cash limit to an ISA.

Generally speaking, there are few restrictions on taking money out. Subject to terms and conditions you can cash in your ISA at any time. And some ISAs, but not all, will allow you to take income. If you want to, you can transfer from one ISA provider to another, but look out for hidden charges, such as exit penalties.

At the time of writing there are **three main types of ISA:**

- Cash ISA
- Investment (stocks and shares) ISA
- Junior ISA

ISAs are popular across the UK. There are 12.5 million adult ISA accounts in the UK, with a total value of about £726 billion. The greatest number of ISA holders are in the 65 and over age group. The split between men and women is approximately equal.[15]

Cash ISAs are the most commonly purchased. They do better when interest rates are high. They are, in effect, savings accounts. They differ from ordinary savings accounts in that you do not have to pay income tax on interest.

Investment (or stocks and shares) ISAs often do better, particularly over the long term, especially when interest rates are low. As with all investments, there is always some risk. Stocks and shares can go up and down, as recent trends have shown.

Most people just buy into a brand-name investment ISA. You should research the performance on a money comparison website before you choose which brand name ISA to invest in.

There are two further ISAs. The Lifetime ISA (LISA) is available for 18–39-year-olds for the purpose of buying a first home or for saving for later life.[16] The Innovative Finance ISA allows you to use your ISA allowance to invest online in 'peer-to-peer lending' (P2P), such as certain types of crowdfunding.

Investing for a grandchild

As always, it is best to take financial advice. There are a whole range of options, depending on how much you wish to give away. You could consider investment funds or money held in trust. You could open an investment account and invest ethically (or otherwise). You could open a personal pension fund or buy Premium Bonds, or just open a bank or building society account.

Many, however, choose a simple option. They pay into a **Junior ISA**, which cannot be touched until the holder is 18 years of age (when it becomes the property of the holder, for them to do with as they wish). Junior ISAs are popular as a way of starting young people saving. They are also recommended by financial advisers as a way for parents or grandparents to give a helping hand. Junior ISAs come free of income tax and capital gains tax. Monthly payments or one-off payments can be made into a Junior ISA, up to £9,000 a year. All ISA limits (which change from time to time) can be found on the HMRC website.

Borrowing Money

Borrowing money can be expensive, but sometimes it becomes necessary.

In later life, you may have substantial costs for your care, particularly if you have live-in carers or other support services at home (whether you own or rent). Understandably, you may well want to stay in your own home as long as you can, or the time may come when you need full-time care which can only be delivered in a care home. For those who have more than modest assets (property, savings and investments), the cost of carers or living in a care home can be expensive. For staying at home, *see pp 232-233*. For costs of care, *see pp 236-242*.

Or you might want to borrow money for repairs to your home, to repay debts, such as a mortgage, or to supplement your pension income. Or you might want to borrow to spend: to provide funds for holidays or luxuries. Or even to pay for the everyday cost of living.

The following are some of the main options.

Equity release

If you own property, it is possible to borrow money against its value.

The **equity** in your home, if you own it outright, is the full value of the property on the open market. But if you have a mortgage or other loan charged against your home, the equity is the value of the property less the mortgage or loan. Equity release is a borrowing scheme, regulated by the Financial Conduct Authority (FCA). It is a scheme by which you can borrow money against the equity.

For more information and general advice on equity release see MoneyHelper, the independent, government-backed money and pension guidance service.[17] The guidance emphasises that you should get professional advice before taking out an equity release product. You may wish to take advice from an Independent Financial Adviser (IFA) who specialises in equity release. It is a specialist subject.

You may also wish to consider an alternative to equity release: downsizing to a smaller (and, perhaps, more manageable) property. This may free up extra capital for your use.

There are two forms of equity release. They both involve your staying in your own home until death or when you have to move out for full-time care. They are both expensive.

- **Lifetime mortgage**
- **Home reversion plan**

Lifetime mortgage

This is the more common of the two forms of equity release. A lifetime mortgage is a **loan secured against the property you own**. The loan will be in the range of 20–60% of the value of the property. You must be at least 55, but at 55 you will only be able to borrow just over 20%. The older you are the more you will be able to borrow. A few companies impose an upper age limit, usually 80 or above.

The loan is received as either:

- one cash lump sum with interest paid from the date of the loan
OR
- as a number of cash lump sums from time to time (eg monthly), with interest paid as and when money is received.

The latter is the cheaper option, but either option is expensive because interest on the loan(s) is **compound interest** (interest upon interest), sometimes called 'rolled-up' interest.

Interest rates for lifetime mortgages vary depending on the current financial situation. They are usually in the range of 5–9%, but have been as low as 4%.

There is a cost to set up the scheme in the range of £1,500–£3,000[18]. This includes fees for set up, valuation of the property and legal fees. There may be extra cost for initial advice.

The loan (the sum borrowed) plus the compound interest is paid back in full from the **proceeds of sale** of the property, on death or on moving out.

I summarise in my own words (*below*) the main advantages and disadvantages of the lifetime mortgage, some of which are informed by MoneyHelper. I considered these when thinking with relatives what might be best for my mother-in-law in her nineties (if and when it came to it).

Home reversion plan

This form of equity release involves the **sale of your home** (or a proportion of your home), which you own, before you move out or die. A home reversion plan involves the sale of the property to a 'reversion provider', such as an insurance company. You must usually be at least 60 years of age.

The reversion provider estimates the value of the property and makes an offer for the property (or a proportion of the property). This offer will be a modest offer, less than the market value (normally 20–60% lower).

If you accept the offer, the reversion provider becomes the owner (or part-owner) of the property. The property is put in their name (or part in their name, part in your name).

The reversion provider benefits from (a) the low purchase price and (b) the increase in value, if any, of the property on your death or moving out.

You get to stay in your home (rent free, usually), with the responsibility for upkeep and maintenance of the property.

As with a lifetime mortgage, there is a cost to set up the scheme of approximately £3,000 (but maybe less). This includes fees for set up, valuation of the property and legal fees. There may be extra cost for initial advice.

I summarise in my own words the main advantages and disadvantages of a home reversion plan, some of which come from MoneyHelper.

There are alternatives to equity release, but they are limited.

The best armour is to keep out of gunshot

Italian proverb

Lifetime Mortgage

ADVANTAGES	DISADVANTAGES
You can stay in your own home (rent free)	Compound interest is very expensive; therefore the shorter the loan (ie as late in life as possible) the better
You will have money to support yourself, maintain your home and pay for any carers	The loan and the interest reduce the value of your estate; there will be less to pass on to your beneficiaries
Interest rates are fixed – you know how much the loan is costing	You continue to remain responsible for the costs of upkeep and maintenance of the property (as per terms and conditions)
You can choose to receive a regular (such as monthly) income, one single lump sum or several smaller lump sums according to your needs	There is a cost to set up the scheme
The risk of 'negative equity' – the estate having to pay the excess if the sale of the property is not enough to repay the loan – can be avoided by a no-negative-equity guarantee (Equity Release Council standard) which most lifetime mortgages offer	When the property is sold, you (or your estate) will be responsible for the costs of the sale
There is no question of repayment (until death or moving out for care purposes)	

Home Reversion Plan

ADVANTAGES	DISADVANTAGES
You can stay in your own home (rent free, usually)	You will receive a lot less than the market value for your home
You will have money to support yourself, maintain your home and pay for any carers	You are no longer the sole owner of your home; you lose the control of being sole owner
You can choose to receive a regular (such as monthly) income, one single lump sum or several smaller lump sums according to your needs	Your estate will be reduced; there will be less to pass on to your beneficiaries
You have the certainty of knowing what proportion of your property you have sold	You continue to remain responsible for the costs of upkeep and maintenance of the property (as per terms and conditions); the reversion provider will regularly inspect the property and you may be bound to carry out repairs which they request
	There is a cost to set up the scheme
	When the property is sold, you (or your estate) will be responsible for the costs of the sale of your remaining (if any) share of the property

Sale and rent back schemes

Avoid them, if possible. They are different to home reversion plans. You sell your home to a private company at a reduced value, then rent it back as a tenant. The rent may be higher than the going market rate and the term of the tenancy may be limited, maybe for five years. After that you may have to leave your home.

Retirement interest-only mortgages (RIOs)

You take out a mortgage in the usual way, a loan charged against your home which you own, and pay back the interest (sometimes even part of the capital) on a monthly basis (during life). You need to have income or other available funds to pay for this option.

The loan is repaid when the term of the loan is completed or when you sell the property or when you die (depending on the terms of the mortgage).

You or your partner or even possibly somebody else such as a beneficiary (for example a close relative) would have to be approved by the mortgage company and assessed by them as capable of keeping up the regular payments (during your life).

This is probably a cheaper option than an equity release lifetime mortgage, because the repayments of the interest are likely to be cheaper as they don't involve compound interest. But, of course, the interest payments have to be made during life, whereas with the equity release lifetime mortgage they do not. It may be a more flexible option, more open to negotiation (or at least discussion) on the terms. And if the interest payments during life are not kept up, your home is at risk of repossession.

As an alternative, a beneficiary under your will or a trusted relative or friend could take out a mortgage charged against their own property. Or they could just lend you the money, if they have sufficient funds, at decent agreed rates, and you alter your will by adding a codicil so that they are repaid out of your estate.

Any other form of loan will also involve repayment instalments during life.

Cash from pension pot

If you have a private pension pot, you may be able to draw down money from it (*see pp 121–122*).

Overdraft or credit card

This is not a good way of borrowing money, except small amounts in the short term. Overdrafts are expensive, unless agreed with the bank for a limited period. Credit cards are expensive too, unless you pay back what you owe in full on a monthly basis, (*see p 89*).

Check your credit rating

If you want to borrow money (equity release, small loan, business loan, mortgage), you can always check your own **credit rating** first. Sign up to one or more of the three main UK credit reference agencies (CRAs): Experian, Equifax and TransUnion.[19]

You will have to answer questions about yourself and your banks before they will tell you your rating. They will check your credit-worthiness by seeing, for example, if you paid off your credit balances promptly over the years, whether you paid bills on time, cancelled a direct debit too quickly, changed addresses and missed a deadline because of a letter not forwarded to your new address, etc. Your detailed credit file is stored ready for you to access (sometimes for a fee). The purpose is to show whether you are likely to be credit-worthy when you try to borrow.

Summary on borrowing for later life

If you want or need to borrow a substantial sum of money, I recommend the following:

- Consider downsizing to a smaller and cheaper property (if you own one) before you consider borrowing
- Take appropriate professional advice (from an FCA regulated adviser); the options you face and the financial implications are far from straightforward

- Get advice tailored precisely to your situation
- Borrow as little as you can, as late as you can; as soon as you borrow, the cost of interest becomes expensive; the best deals (the least costly deals) tend to be available to older borrowers
- Try and work out what everything is likely to cost in advance
- Check fees and charges in advance
- Check whether your income tax bill will be affected
- Check whether any benefits you receive are affected

*Spend and be free,
but make no waste*

English proverb

Outgoings

Check your regular (or irregular) outgoings.

Check that long-standing direct debits are still wanted. Check for payments for products or services you no longer use or want. For example, you may have signed up for repair insurance for white goods you no longer have. You should, of course, be encouraged to go to the gym. But if you don't and don't want to, you might like to think about not paying for not going. You may still be paying a subscription for a magazine you never read anymore.

If you do cancel a standing order or direct debit, make sure you notify the company providing the product or service in writing. Check that there is no notice period (or fee) for cancellation (as there usually is with gyms). If there is a notice period you will have to comply with it, unless you have special reasons for cancellation. Check out the companies you have never heard of (or can't remember) on your bank or credit card statements, to see what they are, they could be insurance you no longer need.

If there is something on your bank statement you don't understand, such as an abbreviation of REV or TFR, make an online search or get help from the MoneySavingExpert free guide to bank statement codes and abbreviations (and much more). Your bank's website will help, too.

Check your bank statements and credit card statements regularly, for false or misplaced entries. For example, one scam involves regular payments supposedly to well-known insurance companies. If you don't check closely, they can look like proper payments. Check regularly, maybe every day or every week. If something is not right, the bank needs to be informed as soon as possible (*see p 173*).

Once you have a handle on your outgoings, it may be time to look at reducing them – there are many obvious ways to save money by doing this.

Switch

There may be quite a few utility providers, insurance companies, broadband providers and other organisations that you pay money to on a regular basis. You stay with them because you are used to them and don't check every year at the time of renewal. You are a loyal customer.

But if you have stayed with a company or organisation for a long time, you may be suffering a 'loyalty penalty'. This means that you are being charged more than you should be because you don't shop around. You just stay comfortably, but less profitably, where you are. This affects 'loyal' older people particularly. New customers often get better deals.

If you **switch** from one provider to another you may get a better deal. The money comparison websites will help you get the best deal.[20] If you phone your company shortly before annual renewal, you may get a better deal, especially if you tell them what reduction is available if you switch.

Here are a few examples, suggesting possible ways for saving money.

Prudence is a presumption of the future, contracted from experience of time past

Thomas Hobbes, *Leviathan* (1651)

Bank and building society accounts

Money squirreled away in rainy-day savings accounts that earn practically no interest, especially at High Street banks, can be switched to a more profitable account or an ISA. Even though interest rates are often low, there are plenty of better deals around, if you look. Newspapers and money websites suggest the best offers available.

If you have time (and energy) take advantage of the short-term or introductory offers with some banks and building societies, especially online. You may have to move your money again after 12 months, to keep taking advantage of the best offers. But the difference, at times of low interest rates, between 0.5% and 2% interest (or more) can be significant for savings.

If you want to switch to a different bank, consider using the relatively painless and free service at CASS, the current account switch service.[21] Advantages of switching may include better interest rates, a cash bonus, a bank with a branch near you, and better customer service. The switch, involving moving money, direct debits and standing orders, should be completed through CASS within seven days.

Utility providers

You can switch certain utility providers – electricity, gas, broadband and phones – in order to get the best deal. This is not as difficult as it sounds, although in times of energy crisis this may become more difficult because there are likely to be fewer deals. See websites which will help you switch, for example, Uswitch, Energy Helpline, MoneySavingExpert and look at the comparison websites.

There are other commercial sites. They may not charge you, but they may receive a commission from the provider when you 'flip' to a new service provider. After all, they do exist in order to make a profit. And the provider they suggest may not necessarily be the cheapest deal around. You may have to look around and make your own comparisons.

And have you checked your landline phone bill recently (if you still have one)? What exactly are they charging you for? When did you last check or discuss a reduction with them? New customers often pay less than the old ones. Is it time to switch? Or at least, is it time to ring them up and see what deal, what new contract, is on offer? It may be laborious, but it should save you money.

You could use your mobile phone and cancel your landline. You could consider a wifi deal with your TV and landline combined (even if you don't use your landline).

Insurance companies

You may have property or contents insurance. You may have car insurance. Watch out for creeping renewal prices.

The **'loyalty penalty'** (or 'price walking') has been hard at work in the insurance industry over the years, and at the customer's expense. Citizens Advice estimated in 2017 that nearly 13 million householders may have paid a 'loyalty penalty' for their home insurance, some 63% of the insurance market. And 32% of them were over 65. According to Citizens Advice those most likely to be overcharged for staying loyal were the old and the vulnerable.[22]

In January 2022, the Financial Conduct Authority (FCA) banned 'loyalty penalties' in the home and car insurance markets.[23] They are no longer permitted to offer different (and better) prices to new customers than they offer to existing customers. Unfortunately, some ways of getting round this restriction with 're-arrangement' fees or 'set-up' or 'administration' fees have been observed. Other markets, however, still suffer from the loyalty penalty: broadband, mobiles and mortgages.[24]

The customer's options for keeping down creeping annual increases to a reasonable amount are:

- negotiate each year over your existing policy at the time of renewal
- negotiate a new policy, a new contract, with your existing provider (often, as a 'new' customer, with a sign-up discount for a limited period)
- switch to a different provider: cancel the old policy, having looked around for comparison prices, and sign up with a different company

This is all hard work, but, sadly, necessary in order to keep bills down. Make sure you are not losing some aspects of protection, particularly with home insurance, by switching to a cheaper provider. Work out what you want and check the details. According to research, insurance policies are so complicated that almost nine out of ten people cannot understand them.[25] Call companies up and see what they can offer. As I have found with car insurance, they may even ask you what comparisons you have found, and make you an offer.

And don't forget to notify the insurance company of any changes, such as home improvements or a new garden office, even a large cat flap. If you don't, your policy might be null and void. On the other hand, you might even get a reduced premium, for example with a new smart doorbell or a smart heating system.

Credit card debt

If you have debt on your credit card, which can be very expensive, you can sometimes switch to another card provider (*see pp 90–91*).

Haggling

You can always try haggling. If you've got the nerve (and the confidence), have a go. It is surprising what deals can be done. A friend of mine (who used to sell second-hand cars) used to haggle over absolutely everything. He once tried to haggle down the cost of a washing machine in a well-known department store. A rather snooty salesman responded: 'This is Harrods, sir, not the Portobello Road.'

Pay Your Bills (If You Can)

That may be obvious. But if you are struggling to pay bills, **don't delay or ignore**. Take advice, for example from your local Citizens Advice. Renegotiate a payment plan over a longer period (although that may cost more).

There are also movements and campaigns that from time to time encourage people to refuse to pay bills, particularly energy bills. Dontpay.uk, for example, which described itself as 'a grassroots movement demanding a fair price for energy for everyone', invited people in 2022 to pledge to withhold payment when they reached one million pledges. It claimed its campaign (despite not reaching that number) led to results including the energy bill price cap in the winter of 2022.

This may sound fine and high-minded, to battle with increasingly large bills and take a stance, but some charities warn of the consequences of not paying an energy bill.

Let us take gas as an example. This is not a national service. You have entered into a contract with your gas supplier. Not paying your bill will be a breach of contract. What happens if you decide to cancel your direct debit payments? Something like this:

1. Your gas may become more expensive. Paying by direct debit is usually the cheapest method of payment. If you stop your direct debit payments, the price may go up.
2. Your supplier will contact you to discuss a new payment plan, not paying less overall for your gas, just paying it over a longer time with reduced direct debit payments.
3. If you refuse to agree a new payment plan, the supplier may require you to have a pre-payment meter installed (usually more expensive).
4. The supplier may charge extra fees for late payments.
5. After that, disconnection may be a possibility, but only as a last resort; there can be no disconnection between 1 October and 31 March of any year if you are over the State Pension age of 66 and you live alone, with other people over 66, or with children under 18.
6. Your details could be passed to a debt collection agency. There could be charges for this and you may receive 'threatening' letters or calls from the agency (who are not always charming and understanding). They can 'doorstep' you, but they are not bailiffs and cannot seize your property. They can, however, take you to court for non-payment.
7. Your credit rating could be damaged.

Reducing your energy bills

At the time of the energy bill crisis that developed in 2022, many suggestions were made for using less energy at home. Some, apparently, are more successful than others. The Energy Saving Trust,[26] an independent expert on recommending effective energy choices, suggested the top five biggest savings would come from:

- draught-proofing gaps around doors and windows
- reducing your shower time to four minutes (and not having baths)
- insulating your hot-water cylinder
- using your washing machine on a 30-degree cycle, no hotter, and avoiding using a tumble dryer
- turning your electrical appliances (particularly older ones) off standby mode: switching off at the plug socket

Pay your tax on time

If you have tax to pay – income tax, Capital Gains Tax, Stamp Duty or Inheritance Tax – make sure it is paid on time. HMRC charges interest for late payment, at the rate of Bank of England base rate plus 2.5%. If by chance you overpay, HMRC will pay back base rate minus 1%.[27]

If you pay outstanding income tax under a tax debt repayment scheme known as a Time to Pay Arrangement,[28] interest will increase significantly in times of high interest payments. Avoid this form of payment, if you can, or try and renegotiate with HMRC. Late tax penalties will also be affected by higher rates.

Banking

It is still possible to get to a bank near you. Or is it? Banks have closed two thirds of their branches in the last 30 years.[29] How many of them are now coffee shops? One older man, as reported by ITV News, was scammed by a bitcoin investment fraud in 2024. He said that he might have been saved from the scam if his local bank branch had not closed; he would have popped in to speak to the staff who knew him to discuss the investment.

So you really need to get computerised or download your bank's app (with or without help from a trusted younger person). Otherwise you may suffer what is now known as 'digital exclusion'.

Using an app means you will be able to check your bank account and credit card details instantly. You should be doing this on a weekly if not daily basis anyway, to check that nothing is going wrong – no scam payments or dubious withdrawals or incorrect banking charges (*see pp 149, 151–153, 156, 173*).

With the increase of online shopping, particularly for all our daily needs and at busy times like Christmas, there is all the more reason to check your bank accounts regularly.

And as I said earlier in this chapter, do think about your money in those bank accounts that sit around earning next to nothing, particularly when interest rates are on the rise. If you want to earn a little money, you have to shop around for the best deals in savings accounts, whether with ready access or not, depending on your needs (*see also ISAs, above*).

Cash

Over three million consumers are said to rely on cash, most of them being over 65.[30] But the use of cash has fallen dramatically from 62% of all payments in 2006 to 12% of all payments in 2023. One forecast projects a fall to 6% by 2033.[31]

While bank branches have continued to close, ATM availability has declined too. The number of free-to-use ATMs in the UK peaked in 2017 at 55,000, but fell to under 40,000 in 2023.[32]

Nevertheless, if you prefer to use cash, you have the right under the law to have access to a cash service free-of-charge.

In 2023 a new law, designed to provide greater protection for access to cash deposit and withdrawal services, was introduced. The government directed that if you live in an urban area of the UK you should have access to a cash access service, such as a bank, building society or ATM, within a maximum of one mile from where you live. If you live in a rural area, the maximum distance is three miles. The Financial Conduct Authority is required to monitor coverage of these cash services.[33]

In making this policy the government recognised that 'digital payments may not yet be a suitable option for many people who still rely on notes and coins, for example to manage their finances, do their shopping, or to help out friends and relatives'.[34] 'Not yet', anyway.

Personal ID

More and more these days, banks and other financial institutions (and others) require personal ID (identification). We don't (yet) have national ID cards like some countries, although I still have my National Registration Identity Card from October 1946, with the signature of my mother as parent. So a passport and driving licence, both with photos, are the most common form of acceptable photo ID today. Make sure you keep to hand an ID document which is in date for this purpose. For voting ID, *see p 269*.

Some banks also require validation ID (an OTP, a one-time passcode) through a mobile phone number (not a landline) or an email address. There is not a lot you can do about this. If it is a condition of opening an account, you will have to comply. (Someone I know made up a phone number and the bank never queried it. Not something I recommend.) If it is an existing account you may want to argue the toss. But the requirement is becoming more common. For the growing use of Multiple Factor Authentication (MFA, also called two-factor or two-step authentication or 2FA), in which two or more pieces of identification evidence are provided electronically (*see p 145*). The most common factors are (a) a password or PIN, (b) a digital phone or email address, and (c) fingerprint or facial recognition.

Credit and debit cards

A **credit card** lets you spend money on credit. It is as if you are lent the money for each purchase you make with the card. The lender is a bank or other financial institution or other lender. They lend you – the borrower – money which you have to pay back. There will be a pre-set limit as to how much you can borrow.

As the borrower you must pay back the money you have been lent. If you pay back what you have borrowed in full each month, there will be no extra cost. But if you pay back just the minimum required each month, you will be charged interest, and at an expensive rate of repayment. Late payments can be costly too. The easiest way to repay is to set up a direct debit for the full amount you have borrowed every month.

By contrast a **debit card** makes a direct link to your bank account. When you spend with the card, the amount comes straight out of your account. The card will not work if you do not have money in your account or an overdraft facility (which can be expensive).

Paying by credit card: advantages

There are some positive advantages in using a credit card sometimes rather than a debit card. If you pay in advance of delivery for a high-price item such as a bed or a sofa, use a credit card. That provides the best protection for your money if things go wrong. Even if you are just putting down a deposit, use a credit card.

The reason for this is that credit card providers are jointly liable for the goods or service you are paying for in the event of **misrepresentation** or **breach of contract**. If you have a claim against the supplier of the goods you also have a claim against the credit card company (even if you have exceeded your credit) and it may be easier to claim against the credit card company. They have to refund you if the firm goes broke or if you have been cheated or if the retailer/trader fails to deliver (and won't answer your complaints).

This is known as **'section 75' protection:** sections 75 and 75A of the Consumer Credit Act 1974. It applies in all four nations of the UK.

What does section 75 protection cover? It covers goods or services which cost over £100 but no more than £30,000. It also applies to goods due to be supplied to you in the UK but supplied from outside the UK (even purchased outside the UK) and bought online, by telephone or mail order for delivery to the UK.[35]

Section 75A may also cover you if you pay by credit card for goods costing over £30,000 and the credit is up to £60,260, if you have a claim against the supplier but the supplier does not respond, cannot be traced or is insolvent. In those circumstances you may claim against the credit card company (although a Section 75A claim is less straightforward than a section 75 claim).

But section 75 only covers you if you have paid the company **directly** and not through a third party (known as a 'debtor-creditor-supplier agreement'). Payment through a third party includes payment via PayPal (in some circumstances) and other marketplace intermediaries. And if, for example, you booked your holiday or theatre tickets through an agency and something goes wrong, the card provider may consider this a third-party payment which means you may not get compensation. This is because the direct link with the airline or travel company or theatre may have been broken.

If you want protection cover for a substantial purchase, buy directly from the supplier using a credit card.

Therefore, if you buy with a debit card or with cash (or by cheque) you may lose out. Section 75 protection does not apply, although, more commonly now, an exception may apply in the case of debit cards through **chargeback**, a voluntary scheme provided by some but not all debit-card issuers. When a well-known and well-respected bed company suddenly went bust, customers who had ordered a bed **and** paid for it (but not received it) could only guarantee to get their money back if they had paid with a credit card.

Note that credit card companies don't like having to pay up, so be prepared to be persistent.

If you pay partly by credit card, eg for the deposit (even if under £100), and the rest by cash or cheque, you will still be covered for the whole amount.

This is a positive advantage of using a credit card. Other possible advantages include reward schemes such as points or airmiles. You will also improve your credit rating, for example if you later want to apply for a loan or a mortgage, if you buy with your credit card and pay off at the rate agreed, usually in your monthly payment.

Even if your purchase is not section 75 protected, you still have other rights, for example if the goods are faulty or the service agreed is inadequate or the terms of the contract are unfair: see the Consumer Credit Act 2015.

Paying by credit card: disadvantages

You will, however, score badly on your credit rating if you fail to pay off the debt on the credit card or fail to keep up with monthly payments in full. A poor credit rating may affect your chances of applying for a loan or mortgage.

Disadvantages of using a credit card include:

- spending beyond your means and having difficulty paying back the debt
- facing expensive interest charges when you default
- losing out in your credit rating, particularly with banks
- high interest on cash withdrawals
- some lenders charge a fee for the card itself, an initial fee or an annual fee
- some cards are expensive to use overseas

If you are having problems getting a loan or entering into a contract, for example for a phone, you can check with the big three credit rating agencies to find out why (*see p 77*).

*Be not made a beggar by
banqueting upon borrowing*

Ecclesiasticus (c.180 BC)

Credit card debt

The average credit card debt per household in the UK is estimated at more than £2,500.[36] If you have spent beyond your means or for some other reason have built up credit-card debt on one or more cards, you will find it very expensive to repay. As a result, rules were put in place in 2018 to require credit companies to start talking to their customers about persistent debt.[37]

Credit card companies make their money by charging interest, somewhere between 15 and 30%. This is very expensive and soon builds up. Use your credit card wisely. Pay off what you owe by standing order every month. This avoids interest. Paying the monthly minimum repayment and no more is asking for trouble. The interest will grow steeply.

But there is a cheaper way to reduce credit card debt. You can switch your debt from one card to another. Some cards offer a better rate for repayment: 0% **'balance transfer'** deals are offered from time to time, particularly if you have a good credit rating (homeowner, regular employment, etc.). The interest-free periods vary, but they can be as long as 24 months (or even longer).

In this way you can transfer your credit card debt from one card to another, choosing one which charges 0% interest for a fixed period of time. That gives you a bit of a breather, time to pay off some of the debt, without increasing it with high interest-rate charges. This transfer is subject, usually but not always, to a modest 'handling fee', typically a percentage of the debt to be transferred (around 2%). Your repayments of the debt will go towards clearing your outstanding balance and not on interest during that period. So you can clear the debt more quickly, more cheaply.

But take care. If you fail to keep up your monthly repayments or go over your credit limit, the 0% deal could be halted and you would have to face the interest rate, which could be very substantial. So only switch your credit card debt if you are prepared to be disciplined about it. You may want to set up a direct debit to cover at least the minimum payment. You should also note that if your credit rating is poor, your transfer application may be granted on lesser terms or refused altogether.

You should also check the rate that the new card will charge if you are tempted to use it to spend. It could be a high rate. Just when you are trying to reduce debt, the new card's offer can take it away again. Or you can stay with your old card and change to the lowest repayment terms available. But you must keep up the repayments.

If you are unsure about all of this, take advice. Citizens Advice and the debt charity StepChange are very helpful.[38] Citizens Advice recommend dealing with other debts, if you have them, first. They describe them as 'priority debts' such as rent arrears, mortgage arrears, unpaid council tax or utility bills (and much more). If you have debt problems, seek advice urgently. Do not ignore letters threatening eviction or cutting off utility supplies or claiming money.

And just watch out for all those attractive 'easy' monthly payment deals when you buy a sofa or a car. The repayment interest can mount up in a way which is much more expensive than obtaining a loan. These things need to be checked. Just as an overdraft, even one used only rarely, can mount up in charges. It all adds up.

Buy-now-pay-later deals, such as with Klarna, are popular, and can be free of interest, but fees may be charged for missed payments (which may affect your credit rating) and you lose your section 75 protection (although chargeback may be available (*see above*). Some say they can encourage spending beyond your means.

How to deal with credit card debt

- Avoid it by using your credit card wisely – pay the monthly repayments in full by direct debit
- Transfer to a 0% (time restricted) card
- Take advice when debt builds up; don't put your head in the sand

Marriage and Civil Partnership: the Financial Advantages

Marriage is a declining institution. The number of adults married (or in a civil partnership) has fallen below 50% for the first time.[39]

Sir Ken Dodd, the comedian, married his long-term partner, Anne, when he was 90, just two days before his death. There may have been all sorts of reasons for this, not least love and affection. But there would have been clear benefits financially for his new wife on his death. By being married, she could inherit his estate (a very substantial one) free of inheritance tax (IHT). Otherwise, she might have had to pay up to 40% IHT on the bulk of the estate.

There are a number of advantages of being married or in a civil partnership, both legal relationships recognised by the law. For convenience, I will refer to both a married partner and a civil partnership partner as a legal partner. By contrast a so-called 'common-law' husband or wife (in cohabitation), or long-term partner, unmarried and not in a formal civil partnership, is not recognised by the law in these circumstances. They do not generally have the benefit of the common law or any law in this context.

The only points of stage law on which we are all clear are as follows: that if a man dies without leaving a will, then all his property goes to the nearest villain, but if he leaves a will, then all his property goes to whoever can get possession of that will.

Jerome K Jerome, *Stage-Land* (1889)

Wills

If there is no will in place (intestacy), cohabiting partners, unmarried and not in a civil partnership, do not have any rights to their partner's estate. If there is no will, you are likely to inherit nothing. Under the intestacy rules the estate will go to members of your partner's family – children first, then parents and siblings of your partner and other family members. The intestacy rules are set out in the Inheritance (Provision for Family and Dependants) Act 1975, (*see pp 13-14*).

Inheritance tax (IHT)

On death, a legal partner is able to pass assets to the other free of inheritance tax (IHT). The surviving legal partner can therefore inherit all of the other's assets. In addition, the surviving legal partner can inherit the other's nil rate bands of tax-free allowance, giving the survivor a possible total of up to £1 million worth of assets to pass on to their children before any IHT is payable. For details, *see pp 128-133*.

By contrast, the surviving partner of an unmarried couple who inherits their partner's estate may have to pay 40% IHT on all assets valued above £325,000.

Inheriting pensions

Only couples who are married or in a civil partnership are allowed to inherit each other's pensions (or a share of them). The State Pension scheme does not recognise unmarried cohabitants.

Some private and occupational pension schemes do recognise cohabiting partners, but only if the terms of the contract permit it.

Capital Gains Tax (CGT)

Transfers between partners who are married or in a civil partnership are tax neutral. A legal partner can make full use of annual and other CGT exemptions. This does not apply to unmarried partners.

Banking

On death of a partner, the surviving unmarried partner will have no access to the deceased's separate (not joint) bank account. The money in the account belongs to the estate, to be settled on probate. If married or in a civil partnership, the bank may allow the surviving partner to withdraw some money from the account.

Separation (not divorce)

If you are unmarried and separate, even after a long-term relationship, the courts will not treat you as if you were married with the usual starting point of 50:50 for the division of assets. If an unmarried partner has all the assets in their name (including, for example, sole title to the home), the other partner will have to argue that they have secured an interest in the assets by having made a contribution in money or money's worth, which is much more difficult. The law may one day catch up and treat married and unmarried partners in the same way. But not yet.

What is the answer?

The answer to all of this is to marry or enter into a civil partnership and make a will in your legal partner's favour, leaving them the whole estate (or whatever you want to leave). On your death, your legal partner will then inherit the whole estate free of IHT, whatever the size of the estate. What is more, when the surviving legal partner dies, they will pass on to their children (or other 'direct descendants') two nil-rate bands of IHT exemption (and possibly also two residential nil-rate bands), so that the children may not have to pay IHT on anything up to £1 million of the estate. That is a very considerable saving.

As an alternative to marriage or civil partnership – and nearly one quarter of couples who live together (in England and Wales), ie over 5.5 million, are not in either[40] – you could enter into a **cohabitation agreement**, a legal document that formalises arrangements for finances, property and children while you are living together, if you split up, become ill or die.[41] You could also seek to put all assets in joint names, such as a property, if you own one or when you buy one. Some advise taking out life insurance to cover any shortfall caused by the law. In any event, each partner could make a will in the other's favour, otherwise the surviving partner may inherit nothing.[42]

If the arrangements are complicated or the assets substantial, consider taking legal advice. This is not an easy legal area.

Problems and Complaints

If you need advice on pensions, tax or wills, you should seek expert independent advice.

For money problems, you can get expert independent advice from your local Citizens Advice, a free and impartial service since 1939.

If you have a problem with any financial transaction, make sure you complain as quickly as you can.[43] Keep a full record of your complaint and always put it in writing. Be clear and straightforward. Summarise the complaint first, then provide details that matter and which explain the problem.

If you find any unauthorised transaction on your bank account or bank (or other) card, call the bank or card issuer immediately. Any delay on your part may be held against you.

The Financial Ombudsman Service (FOS)

This is a helpful, free and independent service. It was set up by Parliament to resolve individual financial complaints. In 2023–24 the FOS received nearly 200,000 new complaints, claiming a 37% overall uphold rate.[44]

The FOS settles disputes between individuals and businesses that provide financial services. If a business has made a mistake or treated you unfairly, the FOS has power to pay you compensation for financial and non-financial loss up to £430,000.[45]

The consumer watchdog organisation *Which?* lists the common areas of complaint which the FOS deals with as:

- most bank accounts
- investment products
- mortgages
- loans
- some pension products
- PPI (payment protection insurance) claims
- insurance policies
- credit and store cards
- HP (hire purchase) agreements
- financial advice

Typically, says *Which?*, a complaint may be made for an insurance pay-out which is refused, a bank which fails to reimburse you after credit or debit card fraud, or when you are charged incorrectly for a financial service.

According to the FOS itself, current accounts are the most complained about product, with a substantial proportion relating to victims of fraud and scams, most relating to 'authorise' fraud (or 'authorised push payments'), where consumers are tricked into transferring money into accounts they believe are legitimate. There is also an increase in complaints about scams involving social media, fake investments (including investments via a 'crypto-exchange' that does not exist) and scams tricking the customer into handing over bank details (*see pp 145–179*).

The FOS advises that before you take your complaint to them you should contact the business first and give them the opportunity to put things right. You may have to complete the business's internal complaints procedure before making a complaint to the FOS. If still not satisfied, contact the FOS at www.financial-ombudsman.org.uk or call 0800 023 4567. The service is free of charge and therefore much cheaper than going to court. Make sure you complain to the FOS within six months of the firm's final response to your complaint.

If your problem is a pensions problem, you may be referred by the FOS to or you can complain directly to the **Pensions Ombudsman** (*see pp 123–124*).

Advice on money complaints is given on a number of independent websites:

- gov.uk
- The Money Advice Service
- The Financial Ombudsman
- The Pensions Ombudsman
- The Energy Ombudsman
- Citizens Advice

A few years after the financial crisis of 2007–8, the Financial Services Authority (FSA, 2001–13) was disbanded and replaced by the Financial Conduct Authority (FCA, 2013) together with the Prudential Regulation Authority (PRA).

The Financial Conduct Authority (FCA)

This is the UK's official financial regulator. It is the conduct regulator for about 50,000 financial services firms in the UK, see www.fca.org.uk. Among other things, they list the properly 'authorised' firms and individuals in their Financial Services Register: see www.register.fca.org.uk. If, for example, you want to check whether a firm or an individual is a properly 'authorised' Independent Financial Adviser (IFA), with authorisation to provide regulated financial products and services, **check the Register**. Some unauthorised firms are also listed on the Register with prominent warnings.

In July 2023 the FCA also introduced a new Consumer Duty, a set of rules for the financial industry to provide higher standards to customers and greater protection for consumers in the retail financial markets.[46] The duty directs that financial products should be provided in a way which is neither misleading nor difficult to understand. It is also designed to try and stop the sale of products and services that are not right for the individual consumer and that do not offer fair value.

The FCA does not investigate individual complaints. It refers you to the Financial Ombudsman Service (above) if your complaint to the individual, firm or organisation has failed. But the FCA website does help on how best to make a complaint: see *How to complain*.[47]

The FCA also advises *How to claim compensation if a* [regulated] *firm fails*.[48] You may be covered, in part at least, by the **Financial Services Compensation Scheme (FSCS)**, a scheme set up by Parliament and funded by the financial services industry. It is independent and access to the service is free.

If you have savings in a bank or building society (if authorised by the Prudential Regulation Authority, *see below*) that fails, the FSCS will automatically (and usually quickly) compensate you up to a maximum of £85,000 per eligible person, per bank or building society, or up to £170,000 for joint accounts.

The Prudential Regulation Authority (PRA) supervises about 1,500 financial institutions. These include banks, building societies, credit unions, insurance companies and major investment firms. This supervision provides some form of protection for you if the institution fails. The PRA is, for example, responsible for the exercise of the FSCS's functions if a bank or building society fails.

Many newspapers and other organisations have financial complaints pages you can contact, for example the *Financial Times* or *The Times* Money Mentor Troubleshooter or the *Guardian* money pages on Saturdays.

Treat Yourself

Regular treats are something to look forward to: an outing to a restaurant, cinema or theatre; a concert or a gig; a trip somewhere, maybe to the seaside; a meet-up with friends; a shared bottle of wine; a dessert, chocolate or sweets – a pleasure to look forward to (all in moderation, of course).

A little treat goes a long way, both in anticipation and execution. And you can probably afford it. You may even be able to afford a bigger treat: a cruise, a holiday abroad, a trip to Australia to see the grandchildren.

According to financial advisers, their more well-off clients do not always listen to the advice that they should splash out and spend more. It's all very well investing and saving, they say, but you may have accumulated more money than you need, so you should consider spending some more. So, consider a splurge now and then. If not a splurge, consider handing it on or giving it away. While you are benefitting from your wealth (if you have it), why not let others benefit too?

On the other hand, you can see why reluctance to spend can bed in. The cost of care in later life can be huge. We must all anticipate the possibility of a longer, later life. So you must plan for this cost, too, whatever you can afford, and work out how much you can splurge or give away. Take advice. Consider your total pot and what you need, now and in the future.

Whether it is a splurge or a treat, you probably deserve it. After all, it well may be the fruit of a lifetime of honest endeavour.

One of the secrets of a happy life is continuous small treats.

Iris Murdoch, *The Sea, The Sea* (1978)[49]

Top Ten Tips

1	**Look after your money**. Manage it and organise your records (for easy access, for overall planning).
2	**Simplify your financial arrangements** to have greater control
3	**Check pensions and benefits for full entitlement** (*see Chapter 3*)
4	**Make your savings work for you**. Take sound advice.
5	**Check your income against your outgoings** and organise a budget plan (if it suits you)
6	**Consider ways to reduce outgoings** such as switching utility/service providers and insurance companies
7	**In taking financial advice, only trust those who can be safely trusted**, for example a properly regulated (by the FCA) Independent Financial Adviser (IFA)
8	**If you have a debt or money problem, do not ignore it**. Deal with it quickly, don't ignore letters, take advice quickly and avoid credit card debt.
9	**Check bank statements and credit card statements regularly** to check for false (scam) or incorrect entries
10	**Make room for treats** because money isn't just for saving

CHAPTER 3

Pensions and Pension Credit

*When I am an old woman I shall wear purple
With a red hat which doesn't go, and doesn't
  suit me.
And I shall spend my pension on brandy and
  summer gloves
And satin sandals, and say we've got no money
  for butter.*

Jenny Joseph, *Warning* (1961)

For most people, pensions are the major if not the sole source of income in older age. Whether the State Pension, workplace pensions or personal pensions, or a combination, they form the backbone of regular income. It is important to get the best and make the best out of them.

Some of us may work full time or part time in our older years, maybe out of choice. And this may provide an income additional to our pensions. Others do volunteer work or have family duties. But pensions should be there for all of us.

In some cases, benefits are available too, such as Pension Credit and Attendance Allowance.

This chapter will look at the options available and how to make the most of them.

The State Pension

You qualify for a State Pension if:

- you have reached the State Pension age, **and**
- you have made contributions (or have sufficient credits) for the right number of years

The State Pension is not means-tested. It is taxable income. It applies to all four countries of the UK.

The State Pension age

Everyone who qualifies is entitled to a State Pension at the age of 66. This is the universal State Pension age, the same for men and women. To qualify you have to have made the required National Insurance contributions through work, whether employed or self-employed, or have sufficient National Insurance Credits (*see pp 104–105*).

State Pension: date of actual and proposed age increases	Age	Universal (from November 2018)
From October 2020[1]	66	Men and women
Sometime between 2026 and 2028[2]	67	Men and women
Currently, sometime between 2044 and 2046 (but subject to review)[3]	68	Men and women

These figures are based upon the Pensions Acts 2007 and 2014 and as discussed in the government *Independent Reviews of the State Pension Age* in 2017 and 2023.[4] The Pensions Act 2014 requires governments to review the State Pension age. The changes reflect expected changes in life expectancy. These age targets may, however, be changed in the future. There is constant pressure on governments to reduce the ever-increasing cost of pensions and benefits.

The largest source of annually managed public expenditure is the social security budget, with pensioner spending[5] as the single largest item. This accounts for over 40% of that budget, about 11.5% of total public spending, amounting annually to more than £125 billion on state pensions alone.[6] The number of pension claimants, nearly 13 million, increases year by year and is expected to grow by one third to nearly 17 million people by 2042.[7]

Some have argued that the **target pension age** of 68 is too young. One think-tank has suggested 70 by 2028 and 75 by 2035, arguing that a later pension age would 'better reflect the longer life expectations that we now enjoy'.[8]

Others say that 70 or 75 is too old for the State Pension age, particularly for those involved in manual or physical work including those in public service such as firefighters, paramedics and prison officers. They argue that pensioners have earned their peace of mind and a quiet life well before 75, if not before 70.[9] They should receive their return on National Insurance contributions paid over many years. And in some areas, such as Blackpool (with a higher than the national average population in the 65 and over age group), life expectancy for men is less than 75 anyway.[10] There could be no return at all.

It has been estimated that about 500,000 people aged over 70 were in full or part-time employment in 2019 (pre-pandemic). That suggests that one in twelve people in their seventies are working (compared with one in 22 some ten years before).[11] It also means that 11 out of 12 are not working, choosing to draw their pension.

Retirement age varies in different countries. In France, for example, the age was 62, one of the lowest in Europe. In 2022 President Macron faced the possibility of nation-wide strikes and disorder, after his declared intention to increase the age to 65 (in order to increase productivity). In the end, 64 was the compromise age. Some European countries have higher retirement ages than France, for example[12]:

- UK, Ireland, Germany: 66
- Portugal: 66.4
- Spain: 66.6
- Italy, Denmark, Norway, Iceland, Greece, Netherlands: 67

The old and the new State Pension

The current State Pension is called the new State Pension or the new 'single tier' (flat rate) pension, with a single weekly payment. It applies to those of pensionable age who were born on or after 6 April 1957 (men) or 6 April 1953 (women).

This replaced the previous two-tier system (basic rate plus additional rate). But the old State Pension for those born before the above dates is still in force (with the Additional State Pension added automatically, if eligible). It is called the old or basic State Pension. Confusingly, the new State Pension is also referred to sometimes as the new basic State Pension.

The new pension was introduced in April 2016 with a view to making the State Pension simpler. But it is still far from simple. This chapter is only a guide. If in doubt as to your eligibility and entitlement, take expert advice.

Qualification: payment contributions (or credits)

You are entitled to the full new State Pension if you have reached the qualifying age of 66 **and** you have a total of **35 qualifying years** of National Insurance contributions or credits. This means[13] you were either:

- working and making National Insurance contributions, or
- making voluntary National Insurance contributions, or
- getting National Insurance Credits, for example for unemployment, sickness or as a parent or carer

The minimum number of qualifying years is currently 10 years, the maximum 35 years. It has not always been 35 years. The latest periods were brought into force in 2016, affecting people who have retired since then. The table below sets out the number of required qualifying years based on different dates of birth

If you have at least 10 years' contributions but fewer than 35 qualifying years (because you have had, for example, career breaks), your basic State Pension will be proportionately less than the full weekly payment, although you might be able to top up by paying voluntary National Insurance contributions.[14]

Working people do not pay National Insurance contributions when they reach State Pension age, although voluntary contributions for top-up purposes can be made after that age.

WHEN BORN	QUALIFYING YEARS
Man born before 6 April 1945	44
Woman born before 6 April 1950	39
Man born 6 April 1945–5 April 1951	30
Woman born 6 April 1950–5 April 1953	30
Man born after 5 April 1951	**35**
Woman born after 5 April 1953	**35**

Check what to expect

You can check with the gov.uk website under *Check your State Pension forecast* to find out how much to expect when you retire: what pension to expect and when, and how to increase it (if you can).

The pensions 'triple-lock'

One aspect of government policy often under threat (because it can be expensive) is the 'triple-lock guarantee'. Despite there being more than 12.5 million pensioners[15] (and increasing), successive governments since 2010 have continued to adhere to the triple-lock pension system, under which State Pensions are increased each year to protect pensioners from inflation. It is based on whichever of the following is the highest of the three:

- the rate of inflation (based on the Consumer Prices Index)
- average earnings growth, or
- 2.5%

In the tax year 2020–21, the average earnings growth was the highest of the three at 3.9%. State Pensions were therefore increased by 3.9%. In 2021–22, the increase was 2.5%. In 2022–23 the increase was 3.1%. In 2023–24 the increase was 10.1%. In 2024–25 the increase was 8.5%. In 2025–26 the increase will be 4.1%, based on 2024's average earnings growth figure.

How safe is the triple-lock 'guarantee'? Despite the pledge in the Conservative manifesto (and in Labour's) before the 2019 General Election to keep the triple-lock, it was 'suspended' for one year in the tax year 2022–23, because of the Covid-19 pandemic. The average earnings increase, at 7.3%, was considered to be too expensive.[16] Instead, the State Pension was increased by 3.1%, the rate of inflation figure.

In June 2022 the Chief Secretary to the Treasury confirmed that the triple-lock would be reinstated for 2023–24, despite the rise in inflation then at over 9%. This was confirmed by the then Chancellor Rishi Sunak who referred to pensioners as being 'among the most vulnerable in society'. This, however, was queried in October 2022 by Prime Minister Liz Truss's second Chancellor Jeremy Hunt, following the reversal of Chancellor Kwasi Kwarteng's 'mini-budget'. But those were uncertain times. Within two days Liz Truss announced that she would keep the triple lock. This was confirmed in the Chancellor Jeremy Hunt's Autumn Statement in 2023 during Rishi Sunak's premiership and confirmed in 2024. Both the Conservative Party and the Labour Party have committed to the triple lock until around the end of the 2020s.

It seems, then, that the triple-lock 'guarantee' is guaranteed for now. But for how long? Although the rate of increase of life expectancy is showing signs of slowing, it is still projected that there will be an extra 5 million pensioners by 2070.[17] Government options, therefore, include abolishing the triple-lock altogether (or putting a cap on it) and/or increasing the state pension age. Both would save the Government a great deal of money, now and in the future.

Payment

For those with the necessary pension contributions (or credits), payment of the State Pension in recent tax years has been as follows:

2021–22	£179.60 pw	£9,339 pa	**New full** State Pension for those reaching State Pension age on or after 6 April 2016
	£137.60	£7,155	**Old full basic** State Pension for those reaching State Pension age before 6 April 2016
2022–23	£185.15	£9,630	New full
	£141.85	£7,373	Basic full
2023–24	£203.85	£10,600	New full
	£156.20	£8,122	Basic full
2024–25	£221.20	£11,502	New full: 8.5% increase
	£169.50	£8,814	Basic full
2025–26	£230.27	£11,974	New full: 4.1% increase
	£176.45	£9,175	Basic full: 4.1% increase

The 2024–25 figure of £221.20 (an increase of 8.5% on the previous year), rising to £230.27 a week in 2025–26 (an increase of 4.1%), for those who reached State Pension age on or after 6 April 2016, is based on at least thirty-five years of NI contributions and/or credits.

The amount of payment per week is dependent on the number of years of contributions. For the full State Pension in 2024–25, for example:

- 35 years of NI contributions and/or credits produced £221.20 pw
- 30 years of NI contributions and/or credits produced £189.60 pw
- 10 years of NI contributions and/or credits produced £63.20 pw

Payment of State Pension is paid on a day of the week according to the last two digits of your National Insurance number.[18]

- 00–19: Monday
- 20–39: Tuesday
- 40–59: Wednesday
- 60–79: Thursday
- 80–99: Friday

Deferment

If you wish, you can defer your State Pension age to a date of your choice. You do not have to do anything; your pension will be automatically deferred until you claim it. In due course you will be entitled to an increased pension amount or the ordinary pension plus a lump sum (for the old state pension only and if deferment is at least one year). You may choose to do this, for example, if you are still working after reaching the qualifying age of 66.

The minimum deferment period is five weeks for the old pension and nine weeks under the new.

Inheriting pensions

In essence, there is a limited possibility of inheriting part of a State Pension or increasing your own State Pension when a spouse or civil partner dies (even if separated). It applies only when those who died were on the old State Pension; they must therefore have reached pension age before 6 April 2016.

Where it applies, any surviving partner (unless they have remarried or entered into a new civil partnership) who has less than a full pension (the old pension) because of not having made sufficient National Insurance (NI) contributions, may have the benefit of the deceased's fuller NI contribution record so as to increase or top up their own pension (up to a maximum of £169.50 in the year 2024–25). This does not apply to surviving partners on the new State Pension.

There may sometimes be payments, too, if the deceased partner received what was called the Additional State Pension (on top of the old State Pension). You should note that there are detailed conditions restricting payment, but where it applies, this will be paid to the surviving partner either now, if pension age has been reached, or when it is reached.

The rules are complicated: always check for any entitlement. Contact the Pension Service.

If the pension of the spouse or civil partner who died was a workplace-defined contribution pension or a personal pension (*see below*), inheriting the pension is more common. Any entitlement to inherit the pension or a part of it will depend on the detail in the pension scheme and on whether the spouse or civil partner was 'nominated' as a beneficiary under the scheme.

There may be income tax to pay on a pension you inherit. If you are on benefits, it may affect your benefits.

Income tax

All pension payments from the government (including a lump sum if you are entitled to one and take it) are paid gross and are subject to income tax.[19] Any income over and above the current personal tax allowance of £12,570 will attract a tax payment. Income in this context includes:

- the state pension
- a workplace pension
- a private pension
- income from any work (employed or self-employed, full-time or part-time)
- any other income, such as money from investments, property or savings

National insurance

Persons of State Pension age, employed or self-employed, full-time or part-time, do not currently pay national insurance (the additional form of income tax for health, care, etc. which is, however, not ring-fenced for those purposes).[20]

In September 2021 the UK Government (Prime Minister Boris Johnson and Chancellor Rishi Sunak) introduced a new tax which was going to affect some pensioners. It was to be called the Health and Social Care Levy (brought into effect by the Health and Social Care Levy Act 2021).[21] The purpose of the Levy, a 1.25% increase in National Insurance (NI) contributions (in the tax year 2022–23), was to provide a substantial increase in funds for the NHS and social care.

The Office for Budget Responsibility estimated that the levy would produce about £12.4 billion a year for ring-fenced health and social care over the three-year period 2022–25.[22] But the NI increase and the levy were scrapped in September 2022 by the short-lived tax-cutting government of Prime Minister Liz Truss and Chancellor Kwasi Kwarteng as from 6 November 2022.[23] As a result, pensioners in employment or self-employed, who would have had to pay towards the levy from April 2023, were absolved from having to make any NI contributions.

The levy has not been reinstated. For details, *see pp 244–245*.

Pension Credit

This applies to those of State Pension age who are living on a low income. You may be entitled to certain extra benefits, on top of your State Pension or if you do not have one. Pension Credit is means-tested and is an income-related benefit.

There are two separate parts to Pension Credit:

- Guarantee Credit
- Savings Credit

You may be entitled to either or both. You must, of course, be of State Pension qualifying age, currently 66 years, and if you are in a couple both of you must be of State Pension age.

Guarantee Credit

This tops up your weekly income to a minimum level, £218.15 for a single person or £332.95 for a couple (2024–25), increasing to £227.09 and £346.60 respectively (2025–26). There are special add-ons if you are a carer or are severely disabled (Severe Disability Addition). If you receive Guarantee Credit you will also be entitled to other benefits such as Housing Benefit and Council Tax Reduction.

Savings Credit

This is the other part of Pension Credit. It is an entitlement to a modest add-on to your pension if you have saved some money towards your retirement. This is also means-tested. Savings Credit is only available if you reached pension age before 6 April 2016. Savings Credit is £17.01 extra per week or £19.04 for a couple (2024–25), rising to £17.70 and £19.82 respectively (2025–26).

Pension Credit is available in all four nations of the UK.

To claim Pension Credit go to gov.uk, *Pension Credit: How to claim* at www.gov.uk/pension-credit; or in Northern Ireland, nidirect.gov.uk, *Understanding Pension Credit*. Or call the Pension Credit claim line on 0800 99 1234; Northern Ireland 0808 100 6165.

Pension Credit was introduced in 2003, replacing the 'minimum income guarantee' and, before that, 'income support' for the over-sixties.[24]

The charity Age UK has long campaigned for the Government to promote greater awareness of Pension Credit.[25] It believes that many less well-off pensioners are missing out on unclaimed benefits. While 1.4 million people receive Pension Credit, MoneySavingExpert has estimated that nearly one million pensioners have failed to claim.[26]

Other benefits

If you are in receipt of Pension Credit (however small), you may be entitled to a range of other benefits and discounts. These include housing benefit, warm home discount, help with dental care and glasses, and free TV licence if you're over 75.[27] You may also claim Council Tax reduction (Council Tax Support), for example, if you live alone and are on low income or Pension Credit.

There are other possible benefits and grants (whether you receive Pension Credit or not), such as:

- Attendance Allowance
- Disability Living Allowance/Personal Independence Payment
- Disabled Facilities Grant
- Carer's allowance (if you care for someone) (*see pp 234–235*)
- Heating benefits
- Transport concessions
- Reduced NHS costs (eg dental treatment, glasses)

Attendance Allowance is a non-means-tested benefit which applies to the over 65s in the UK. Over 1.5 million people claim it.[28] It is tax free. You can claim it if you have a long-term physical or mental illness or disability that means you need help with your daily personal care, such as tasks like washing and dressing. It is paid at two different rates, £72.65 pw, or £108.55 pw (2024–25), rising to £73.88 and £110.39 respectively (2025–26), depending on the level of care you need. The lower rate is for care during either the day or night; the higher rate is for care during both the day and night. Any money received does not have to be spent on care.

Make a claim for Attendance Allowance to the Department of Work and Pensions on a claim form:

Go to gov.uk, *Attendance Allowance*, for Attendance Allowance claim form (Form AA1), or

Call 0800 731 0122 (or 0800 587 0912 in Northern Ireland)

There is a different claim form in Northern Ireland: see nidirect.gov.uk, *Attendance Allowance claim form and guidance*.

An assessment for a claim for Attendance Allowance may in some cases include a visit from a doctor.

Disability Living Allowance is a benefit to help disabled people with care and mobility needs. It is gradually being replaced by the Personal Independence Payment (for those under State Pension age) and the Attendance Allowance.

A Disabled Facilities Grant (DFG) may be available from your council for an adaptation in your home or equipment to help you live safely at home. The Grant is means-tested, but grants can be substantial. Smaller adaptations, such as handrails and lever taps, may be free following a local authority needs assessment (*see p 230*).

Some charities offer help in assessing whether you are entitled to benefits. For example, Independent Age have an online benefits calculator: see independentage.entitledto.co.uk.

Benefits following a death

There used to be a number of limited benefit payments available following a death. They included:

- Bereavement Allowance (formerly Widow's Pension)
- Bereavement Payment
- Widowed Parent's Allowance

These have now all been replaced by **Bereavement Support Payment**[29] (although if you claim Widowed Parent's Allowance, at £148.40 per week,[30] it continues while you remain eligible). This does not apply if you had reached State Pension age at the date of death.

You may be eligible for Bereavement Support Payment, a non-means-tested tax-free benefit, if the following apply:

- your partner (whether married, in a civil partnership or cohabiting with a dependent child under 20) was the person who died
- your partner died on or after 6 April 2017

- your partner had paid sufficient National Insurance payments OR
- your partner died because of a work-related accident or disease
- you are under State Pension age

You should claim as soon as possible, preferably within three months of the death. There are two rates of payment, the maximum being a £3,500 lump sum plus up to 18 monthly payments of £350. You cannot claim if you are divorced, remarried or are in prison.

You may be entitled to the higher rate of this benefit if you were entitled to Child Benefit (or were expecting a child) when your partner died.

See gov.uk, *Apply for Bereavement Support Payment*. Or call the Bereavement Service on 0800 151 2012.

Winter Fuel Payment

For winter 2024–25 (and beyond) the Winter Fuel Payment, which had previously been available to all persons of State Pension age, is restricted to those of State Pension age (or their partner) on Pension Credit or certain means-tested benefits. The current sum is £200 for those aged 66 to 79 or £300 for those aged 80 and over. If you live in a care home or nursing home, the sums are £100 and £150 respectively. If you are a couple only one of you will receive it.[31]

Scotland has made a similar change, applying means-testing to the annual Pension Age Winter Heating Payment. Northern Ireland felt tied to the change in England and Wales and therefore reluctantly followed suit.

For those in the UK of modest means or in hardship, the Warm Home Discount scheme provides a one-off discount of £150 on electricity bills (for Northern Ireland see the Affordable Warmth scheme). Local authorities may also provide help with energy bills through the Household Support Fund (for Northern Ireland see the Finance Support Service). There is also the Cold Weather Payment of £25 for each period of seven days between November and March when the weather falls to zero degrees Celsius. Scotland, separately, has the annual Winter Heating Payment, currently £58.75.

TV licence for over-75s

Free licences for the over-75s were introduced in 1999, but stopped in 2020. They are still free for those 75 and over, but only if you, or your partner living at the same address, are receiving Pension Credit.[32] There are discounts up to 50% if you are registered blind (severely sight impaired).[33]

State Pension and Benefits Checks

Check your entitlement to State Pension. If you are not receiving full pension because you have not made sufficient National Insurance contributions, you may be able to top up by paying voluntary contributions.

See gov.uk website.

Look out for the annual increase under pensions 'triple-lock', if it's still in place.

Check entitlement to Pension Credit if your means are modest.

Check entitlement to other benefits such as Attendance Allowance, which is not means-tested

Workplace Pensions

If you have been employed you may have one or both of the following types of pension through your employer(s):

- a **defined contribution** pension (also known as an occupational or money-purchase pension), by which the money paid in by you and/or your employer is placed in pension investments (like personal pensions, below) and will

provide a pension pot, the size of which depends on how well the investments have done
- a **defined benefit** pension (also known as a **final salary** or career-average pension) which is based on your salary, how long you have worked, and a calculation based on the rules of the specific pension scheme

These pensions and your entitlement are complicated, and so is the language. This is only a summary of some of the key points. You may, for example, have had several employers who have acted in different ways. The government estimates that people have on average 11 employed jobs during their lifetime.

Younger people particularly should check if they are entitled to **'automatic enrolment'**, a government scheme phased in between 2012 and 2018 for those aged 22–65 and earning at least £10,000 p.a. It makes it compulsory for employers to enrol eligible workers automatically in a workplace pension scheme, a scheme which is regulated by The Pensions Regulator (TPR).

Your employer must tell you in writing that you have been enrolled. It is something any employee should take advantage of – a win-win situation: you put money into your workplace pension by your employer taking money out of your pay; your employer is required to add money to it; and (usually) the government also contributes with tax relief. This is a good way of saving for the future.

The gov.uk website, *Workplace Pensions*, gives the following example of how it can work. Each payday £80 goes into your workplace pension:

- you put in £40
- your employer puts in £30
- you get £10 government tax relief

The percentage of your earnings you put into the scheme depends on the pension scheme your employer has chosen.

Some employees who are not eligible for automatic enrolment may have the right to 'opt in' or 'join' a workplace pension. Apply to your employer in writing. You can 'opt in' if:

- you are 16–21 or 66–74, earning above £10,000 pa, or
- you are 16–74, earning between £6,240 and £10,000 pa

You can 'join' if:

- you are 16–74, earning £6,240 or less pa

There is a difference between opting in and joining. If you are able to 'opt in' to a workplace pension scheme, your employer must make contributions (which adds to your pension). If you 'join' a workplace pension scheme, your employer does not have to make contributions, but may do so voluntarily. See The Pensions Regulator, *Opting in and joining*.

It is estimated that over £400 million is sitting in **lost pensions**, waiting to be reclaimed. If you are not sure whether you are or were entitled to a workplace pension, you can contact the Government's Pension Tracing Service or the gov.uk service, *Find pension contact details*, but only to obtain contact details. Neither route will lead to your finding out directly whether you have a pension or not.[34]

If you are 50 or over and have a defined contribution (DC) pension, you can get a free Pension Wise appointment with an independent pension specialist to talk about the options for taking your pension money and how each option is taxed. If you have a defined benefit (DB) pension you can get free independent guidance from MoneyHelper by phone on 0800 011 3797 or use their webchat.

As with personal pensions, below, if you have a defined contribution pension pot, you can access it at the age of 55 (rising to 57 in April 2028); 25% can be taken tax free, up to a current limit of £268,275. For this and other options, *see p 120*.

If you're uncertain about your pension entitlement, you can also seek independent financial advice from an approved pensions expert.

It is hoped that a national Pension Dashboards service will also be available in due course to let you see what pensions you have and how much you have saved (*see pp 124–125*).

Personal Pensions

A personal (or private) pension is a pension you organise yourself. It is a contract between a person and a pension provider, often an insurance company. Under the terms of the contract you make payments into the pension scheme (usually regular payments) which are then invested on your behalf. What you get from your pension pot in later life depends how much you put in and how well the investments made on your behalf do.

This is similar to a defined contribution workplace pension, the only differences being you arrange a personal pension yourself (nothing to do with work) and have complete control over it, whereas a defined contribution workplace pension is very much organised by your employer and also has the added benefits for you of contributions from your employer and tax relief (**see above**). You may achieve more by putting money into a workplace pension, if your employer's scheme permits it, and reaping the benefit of those added advantages.

If you are self-employed you will, of course, have no workplace scheme to join, nor a final salary workplace pension to look forward to. You therefore need to consider very seriously joining a personal pension scheme or schemes, so that you have income in later years additional to your State Pension.

This can be complex territory. Even the government's own guidance website has described there being 'low levels of confidence regarding the pensions landscape as a whole'.[35] According to the UK Census 2021, 53% of adults under pension age are contributing to private pensions.

At the date of retirement, as agreed under the personal pension contract, you have options (as with a defined contribution workplace pension) including:

- taking a lump sum, or
- receiving a regular income known as an annuity, or
- a combination of the two

For *options on retirement*, **see below**. The terms of the contract are often called a personal pension plan.

There are plenty of choices if you want to start a pension. There are one-off packages helping you create a financial plan. Or there are plenty of more straightforward pension schemes online. You just join a scheme (which will be an investment scheme) and make a monthly contribution and that's that; you have started saving for your retirement.[36] You can set up a pension at any age, but the sooner you start the better. Make it a habit. Remember that there are tax relief advantages: for every 80p you invest, the government turns it into £1 (for basic rate taxpayers).[37] Or if you have more substantial assets to invest, at least £50,000 (maybe more), you can consult a carefully chosen financial adviser (*see pp 62-65*).

With your pension scheme you can choose the type of investments, such as 'green' options. Or you can leave it to the discretion of the pension provider (or financial adviser). Like all investments, the amount of money in your pension scheme, often called the pension pot, goes up and down (hopefully up) depending on how well the investments do and the risk level which has been agreed under the contract. The size of the final pot will also, of course, depend in the end upon the amount of money you invest and the number of years you invest.

The age of retirement and the date when you can draw from the pot (the pension benefits) depends upon what you have agreed under the contract. The current normal minimum pension age (NMPA) is fifty-five, rising to fifty-seven in April 2028.

You can have more than one scheme. It is sometimes said that a self-employed person should put aside at least one third of earnings in order to maintain the same standard of living in retirement. (The tax-free pensions allowance is currently £60,000.)[38] And who is to say what the State Pension will be and who will be entitled to it in 30 or 40 years?

It is sometimes said that if you divide your private pension savings by about 20, you can estimate roughly how much income it will provide in retirement. £100,000, for example, will produce about £5,000 per year (on top of your State Pension).[39]

To trace any lost pension, whether your own personal pension or from the workplace, contact the Government's free Pension Tracing Service to try and obtain contact details. Phone 0800 731 0193.

Your pension pot: options on retirement

If you have accumulated a pension pot from one or more private pensions or a defined contribution pension from your employer and you have reached the retirement age specified or agreed in the pension contract, you can usually take any of the following options:

- you can do nothing, just leave the pension money until you are ready for it
- you can take an annual payment (income), known as an **annuity**, for the rest of your life
- you can take out an annuity for a fixed term, say five years, to cover the period until you are entitled to your State Pension or the benefits from an occupational final salary scheme
- you can keep your fund invested but take income from the pot, known as Flexi-Access Drawdown (FAD)
- you can cash in all of your pension pot, in which case the first 25% is tax free (meaning, watch out, because the other 75% is taxable income)
- you can cash in smaller sums from time to time, with the first 25% of each sum tax free
- you can take a lump sum to start with, with a smaller annuity as well
- you could combine two or more pensions at retirement to see if this will produce a higher level of income

These choices are not always straightforward. It may be that a combination suits your needs best. It is sensible to take independent financial advice. You should watch out on the tax front too. For example, by increasing your income, you could be taking yourself into a higher income tax bracket.

An annuity: taking a fixed annual sum

For years, if not decades, the annual income from an annuity was the standard option. The annuity would not seem like a lot compared to the money invested in the private pension plan, but it was steady, regular income for later life. And in some contracts, the income continues to be provided for dependants after death.

There is also a variation on this called 'income drawdown', which permits taking income (without an annuity) while still investing the remaining money left in the pot.

A drawdown: taking a lump sum

In 2015 the pension rules changed. Since then, if you are aged 55 or over, you have been able to take out all or part of your pension pot (known as the 'pension commencement lump sum') as a lump sum. The first 25% is tax free, but the rest is taxable as income tax.[40]

The Government was in fact surprised how much tax this change generated. HMRC data shows that by 2024 more than £83.5 billion had been taken from pension pots since 2015 as taxable payments.[41]

This became an attractive option for many older people (those in the 55–59 age bracket have used it most). Suddenly there was so-called 'pension freedom'. You could draw down as much as you liked, when you liked. You could take a luxury holiday, buy a new car, pay off debts, pay off the mortgage, put down a deposit towards a bigger house or do up the existing one, give the money away, even take the cash and re-invest it yourself in the hope that it would provide a better income than the annuity would.

But there are **risks**. When this provision first came into force, pension savers were advised not to go and spend large sums while still in their fifties, leaving a big hole in their financial future. Drawdown investors are now also warned against companies providing poor advice, sometimes unscrupulous and expensive advice (with hidden charges). There is also advice to always ask what a transaction would cost, what financial advice would cost. Some companies carrying out this service have now left the market, ceasing pension transfer activities altogether, after the Pensions Regulator uncovered problems with their advice.

There are scams too (*see Chapter 5*). Reports of pension scams to Action Fraud have increased significantly, with an average loss to each victim of £75,000.[42]

Pension savers are also reminded of the tax implications of increased income (beyond the first 25%).

On the positive side, this form of income drawdown (known officially as 'flexi-access drawdown') has become a popular option. But you need sound advice about the consequences.

On the negative side there may be risks. Some people have been encouraged to spend too early and too freely, when they may have 30 years life ahead of them and may need the cash for care in older age.

The Lump Sum Drawdown

	Advantages	Disadvantages
1	Freedom of choice, giving intelligent pension-savers more financial options in their retirement years	Spending money that could have been kept safely for costly care provision in later life
2	Flexibility: taking (different) amounts out as and when required	Avoiding reliability: a steady, guaranteed income year by year
3	Sensible freeing up of cash for reasonable purposes, having taken sound professional advice	Investing the cash afresh, when leaving it untouched might have earned more – there will be no going back
4	The opportunity for pensioners to buy more flexible (if riskier) pension products	Making poor (risky) decisions without good advice, or taking advice with costly charges and fee structures
5	Avoiding the low-value returns of an annuity	Investing with unscrupulous 'advisers'
6		Liability to increased income tax

Pension Guidance

The **Money and Pensions Service** (MaPS at maps.org.uk) is an independent government-backed service. It provides pension guidance, as well as money and debt guidance, to the public. They call it 'guidance' not 'advice', because they are not allowed to advise you what options to take. (Nor am I.)

This service merged three separate independent services into one organisation in 2019:

- The Pensions Advisory Service (TPAS)
- Pension Wise
- The Money Advice Service (MAS).

The advice that all three provided can now be found at moneyhelper.org.uk, an impartial practical service that is backed by government, which is described as the 'consumer-facing service' of MaPS.

General advice on pensions can be found at **Pension Wise,** which is now part of MoneyHelper.

The **Financial Conduct Authority** (FCA) provides a register of firms, individuals and other bodies that are authorised by them or by the Prudential Regulation Authority (PRA): see fca.org.uk/firms/financial-services-register. The FCA also provides names of unauthorised firms who have been giving advice without the correct authorisation or deliberately running scams.

Advice on locating lost pensions can be found at The Pension Tracing Service (0800 73 0193). See also gov.uk, *Find pension contact details,* for workplace and personal pensions.

Pension Complaints

If you have a problem with a pension product you can complain to the **Pensions Ombudsman** at www.pensions-ombudsman.org.uk. The Pensions Ombudsman is an independent, government-supported service that has legal power to resolve complaints about workplace and personal pensions. First, you should try and resolve the problem yourself, with the company that advised you or the company that sold you the product. But if you are not able to, contact this service.

The **Financial Services Compensation Scheme (FSCS)** may compensate you for a failed private pension scheme or failed pension adviser. Generally, you are protected if the pension was provided by a UK-regulated insurer[43] and if the pension qualifies as a 'contract of long-term insurance', for example an annuity. For more details see www.fscs.org.uk.

The FSCS does not protect against occupational pension schemes (defined benefit pensions) which fail. But compensation may be obtained from the Pension Protection Fund (PPF), an independent Government agency, at www.ppf.co.uk. If an employer becomes insolvent, the PPF is the safety net.

Any other financial complaint may be taken to the Financial Ombudsman Service which has wide legal powers (*see pp 95-96*).

A Pensions Dashboard?

The dashboard idea, which dates back many years as a concept, is that people will be able to see all their pensions online, and securely, in one place.[44] The dashboard will be run by a coalition of state and commercial organisations, including insurers and banks. See pensionsdashboardsprogramme.org.uk.

But the idea has not yet come to fruition. In 2016 the UK Government indicated that a pensions dashboard would be launched by 2019. In 2019 the Government confirmed their intentions, following a consultation.[45] In 2022 the government published and consulted on draft regulations.[46] Trustees and managers of pension schemes were invited to make sure their data was ready.[47] But the commencement of the scheme is not now expected until October 2026, following the development in 2023 of 'a new programme plan' as part of the programme's 'reset activity'.[48]

The Money & Pensions Service (MaPS) will be responsible for the scheme (under the auspices of the DWP).

If and when the pensions dashboard is in place, pension savers will be able to see how much is saved. They will be able to assess whether their pension provisions, including State Pension, workplace pensions and personal pensions, will be sufficient for their retirement years. The dashboard will, in theory at least, let people track the totality of their pensions from multiple sources. Crucially, it will provide people with the opportunity to assess and plan for the future, particularly for retirement.

Top Ten Tips

1. **Keep up your National Insurance contributions** (or credits) for full State Pension entitlement
2. **Check whether you need to top up your contributions and the amount of State Pension you are entitled to** at gov.uk, *Check your State Pension forecast*
3. **Consider deferring receipt of your State Pension** for example, because you are still working. This will increase your State Pension amount.
4. **Check whether you are entitled to benefits.** Some of these, such as Pension Benefit, are means-tested while others, such as Attendance Allowance, are not.
5. **Check your workplace and personal pensions** as you reach retirement, to make sure you obtain full entitlement
6. **Make sure your employer has automatically enrolled you into a pension scheme (if you're eligible).** Automatic enrolled pensions include a 3% employer contribution and a 1% government contribution on top of the 4% deducted from your salary. Check for eligibility at gov.uk, *Workplace pensions*.
7. **Start a personal pension plan.** Pay into it regularly, keep track of it and consider taking expert advice.
8. **Check your pensions on the Pensions Dashboard** when it commences in (possibly) 2026
9. **Look for lost or missing pensions** at the Pension Tracing Service
10. **Keep details of all your pensions (and benefits) together,** either online or in paperwork

CHAPTER 4

Inheritance Tax

A son can bear with equanimity the loss of his father, but the loss of his inheritance may drive him to despair.

Machiavelli, *The Prince* (1513)

Inheritance tax (IHT)

A government tax on the estate (property, money, possessions) of someone who has died

Inheritance tax (IHT) is a tax on a person's estate on death. For IHT purposes, an estate includes property, money, investments, possessions and, potentially, the value of certain gifts made within the seven preceding years (but not inherited pensions until 2027). Inheritance taxation is a technical and complex subject which requires expert tax advice, particularly if you are considering inheritance-tax planning before death. Don't take it from me. I am not an expert and do not pretend to be one.

I shall do no more than summarise the legal ground rules as I understand them and make a few observations. It should also be noted that governments change the rules, rates and criteria from time to time.[1]

The law and practice relating to IHT apply to all four nations of the UK.

More than £7 billion was collected in IHT by HM Revenue & Customs (HMRC) in the tax year 2022–23 (up from £6.1 billion the year before, mainly due to the rise in property prices, and forecast to rise to £7.5 billion in 2024-25), although fewer than 5% of deaths in the UK resulted in an IHT charge.²

Broadly speaking, IHT is charged at 40% on estates valued at more than £325,000. It is payable by the estate after death and before the state grants probate, the process which leads to release of the deceased's assets after payment of debts. For probate, *see pp 286-288*.

The value of an estate worth less than £325,000 is described as being within the 'nil-rate band' and no IHT is charged. The 'nil-rate band' can double to £650,000 if passed on by a spouse or civil partner to the other. It cannot be passed on to an unmarried partner, however long-term the relationship has been (*see pp 137-138*).

Since the figure of £325,000³ – the nil-rate band – is not too far above the average house price in the UK,⁴ the estates of many homeowners will be subject to inheritance tax.

Summary of IHT Rules

IHT is governed in the main by the 278 clauses in the Inheritance Tax Act 1984. The principal IHT rules are in broad terms as follows.

The deceased's estate: nil-rate bands

Above the threshold: IHT is payable as follows:

- On death, IHT is charged on your **estate** only if it is valued above the threshold, namely at **£325,000 or more** in total
- 'Estate' includes property, possessions, money, investments and, potentially, the value of certain gifts made within the seven preceding years (but not inherited pensions until 2027)
- IHT is payable at the rate of 40%
- IHT is due and payable to HMRC *before* probate is granted; probate releases the assets of the estate after any debts and IHT are paid (*see pp 286-288*)

Basic example – no house

The deceased's estate is valued at **£500,000**. The tax-free threshold is **£325,000**. Tax is payable at 40% of **£175,000** (£500,000 less £325,000).

Tax due to HMRC out of the estate is **£70,000**.

The nil-rate band: IHT is **not** payable in the following circumstances.

- Up to **£325,000**-worth of assets is described as the **nil-rate band** and no IHT is charged; IHT is charged only on that part of the estate above that figure, the remaining assets
- A spouse or civil partner can pass on the value of the **unused nil-rate band** to the other so that the surviving person's nil-rate band can double to **£650,000** on their death (but not a partner who is unmarried or not in a civil partnership)
- A spouse or civil partner can also pass on (in their will) the whole estate to the other free of IHT (subject to domicile in the UK)

Inherited pensions, including pension pots, will not be subject to IHT until 2027, although there may be income tax to pay for the beneficiaries. Whether a spouse or civil partner can inherit a workplace or personal pension will depend, not on the deceased's will, but on the terms and conditions in the particular pension schemes (*see p 109*).

The residence nil-rate band (RNRB): IHT is also **not** payable in the following circumstances.

- In addition to the nil-rate band, there is an additional **residence nil-rate band** (or main residence band)[5] for a home (house or flat) left to a spouse or civil partner or 'direct descendants' (such as children, grandchildren, stepchildren, foster children, or spouse or civil partner of the above) – this is currently worth **£175,000**

- IHT is only charged on that part of the estate which exceeds the nil-rate band **plus** the RNRB (i.e. currently £500,000)
- A spouse or civil partner can also pass on the value of the **unused RNRB** to the other so that the surviving person's RNRB can double to £350,000 on their death (but not a partner who is unmarried or not in a civil partnership).

If the deceased had 'downsized' to a smaller house, the estate may qualify for a 'downsizing addition' (IHT allowance), if the former house would have qualified for the RNRB if it had been kept until death. For example, if the deceased moved to a care/nursing home and sold their house to pay for fees there, the estate could still claim the full RNRB.

Basic example – with house

The deceased's estate is valued at **£500,000** (including a house).

The tax-free threshold is £325,000 plus £175,000 (RNRB) i.e. **£500,000**.

£0 tax is payable.

Total nil-rate bands (nil-rate bands plus residence nil-rate bands)

The estate of a person with a residence will be IHT free for the first £325,000 plus a further £175,000 for the residence if it passes to a direct descendant – a total of £500,000. (This is subject to the total estate being valued at less than £2 million. For estates valued at £2 million or over, the residence nil-rate band (RNRB) of £175,000 is reduced for every £1 over £2 million by 50p.)

But even better, this tax-free figure of £500,000 can be doubled. A spouse or civil partner (not an unmarried partner) can pass on to their partner, by passing everything on in their will, £500,000 (their unused nil-rate £325,000 plus their unused residence nil-rate £175,000).

This means that the spouse or civil partner can accrue a total of £1 million tax free for their estate (for example children): their own nil-rate band and residence nil-rate band and their inherited nil-rate band and residence nil-rate band from their spouse or civil partner. Anything above that figure will be taxed at 40%.

The nil-rate band, £325,000, and the residence nil-rate band, £175,000, were fixed in 2022 until 2028 (although can always be changed by Parliament).[6]

Basic example – with house and inherited nil-rate bands

The deceased's estate is valued at **£1,250,000** (including a house).

The tax-free threshold is £325,000 plus £175,000 i.e. £500,000. But the deceased has also inherited by will the same (unused) tax-free threshold from their spouse or civil partner. This doubles the tax-free threshold to **£1 million**.

Tax is payable on the balance of **£250,000** at 40%, i.e. **£100,000**.

Gifts during life

Although it is called inheritance tax, the tax may still be payable on some gifts made during life (sometimes known as gifts *inter vivos*).

Gifts: inheritance tax payable

- Gifts of money during lifetime if you do NOT live for seven years thereafter
- IHT on these non-exempt gifts is charged at 40% on gifts given in the three years before you die; gifts made three to seven years before your death are taxed on a sliding reducing scale known as 'taper relief' (**see below**)[7]

- Gifts in the seven-year period with a combined value of less than £325,000 use up part of the nil-rate band but are not taxable – whatever is left from the nil-rate band is then set against the estate
- Gifts in the seven-year period exceeding £325,000 in value: the excess gifts over and above the nil-rate band are subject to IHT and there would be no remaining nil-rate band to set against the estate

Taper relief for gifts during life

Years between gift and death	% tax to pay
Less than 3	40%
3 to 4	32%
4 to 5	24%
5 to 6	16%
6 to 7	8%
7 or more	0%

On the other hand, some gifts made during life may be free of IHT. They are described as exempt gifts or potentially exempt gifts (PETs).

Exempt gifts: inheritance tax not payable

- **Gifts between spouses** or civil partners. You can give as much as you like during your lifetime, as long as the spouse/partner lives in the UK permanently.
- One gift (to a person not a spouse/civil partner) of **up to £3,000** in any tax year (or several gifts totalling up to £3,000). This is known as the annual exemption. It may be carried forward into the next year to make a gift of or gifts up to £6,000 tax free (but not subsequent years).

- A gift up to the value of £250 each tax year to as many persons as you choose (unless that person has the benefit of another exemption)
- Normal gifts out of income, such as small gifts or for birthdays or Christmas
- Any regular payment out of (excess) income, such as paying rent or mortgage for a child or paying into a savings account for a child under 18 or supporting the living expenses of an elderly relative (so long as the payment leaves you with sufficient income to maintain your usual standard of living)
- Wedding or civil ceremony gifts of up to £1,000 per person (£2,500 for a grandchild or great-grandchild, £5,000 for a child)
- Gifts of both birthday and wedding presents may be made to the same person in the same year

Potentially exempt gifts (PETs)

- Gifts of money during lifetime are free of IHT **if you live for seven years** afterwards. For example, a parent gifting a child cash, say, for a deposit on a property. Should you not survive such a gift by seven years, then these gifts will firstly use up any nil rate band and then potentially become subject to IHT themselves.
- Similarly, a substantial loan e.g. to a child (which may give you more control over the money than a gift); if you later choose to write it off, it becomes a gift (and is exempt from IHT if you live for seven years from the date of the write-off). See also chargeable lifetime transfers, such as a gift into trust for the benefit of a child, which allows some control to be retained over the funds.

Charitable gifts in your will

Leaving a bequest in your will to a charity (or political party) will reduce your estate's IHT liability. Called a 'charitable legacy', it does not count towards the total taxable value of your estate.

Also, if you leave at least 10% of your net estate to charity, it reduces the IHT rate from 40% to 36%.[8]

How to Calculate IHT

The following is a rough guide (no more than a guide) as to how to calculate the IHT to be paid. Some of the detailed rules on pensions which are not set out here may affect the figures.

Step 1 Gross value

Assess gross value of the estate (including the market value of any residential property)

Step 2 Net (IHT taxable) value

In order to arrive at taxable value, deduct from gross value:

- any debts (eg mortgage, funeral costs, solicitor's fees)
- any exempt items (eg gifts to charity)
- any relief items: certain types of assets (eg business or agricultural assets)

Step 3 Available thresholds

Further deduct from gross value any available threshold:

- basic nil-rate band in all cases: £325,000 (less any gifts made within last seven years before death)
- residence nil-rate band: £175,000
- inherited unused nil-rate bands if deceased had inherited from spouse or civil partner in a will: £325,000 + £175,000

Maximum available (all three thresholds): £1,000,000

Step 4 Payment

If final figure is nil or less than nil, pay no IHT

If final figure is more than nil, pay IHT to HMRC: 40% of that final figure

IHT Forms

There are many official HMRC forms relating to IHT: see gov.uk, *Inheritance Tax Forms* (updated July 2020). They include, for example:

- **Form IHT400 Inheritance Tax Account**: this is the main form if there is IHT to pay[9]; in which case you must apply for an Inheritance Tax reference number before submitting this form; in Northern Ireland the relevant form is the Probate Summary, Schedule IHT421; in Scotland this form is the Confirmation form, C1
- Schedule IHT402 Claim to transfer unused nil-rate band
- Schedule IHT406 Bank and building society accounts and National Savings and Investments (only those in deceased's sole name)
- Schedule IHT435 Claim for residence nil-rate band
- Schedule IHT436 Claim to transfer any unused residence nil-rate band

Payment of IHT

Payment of inheritance tax (IHT) is made to HMRC by the person dealing with the deceased's estate: the executor(s), if there is a will; the administrator, if there is no will, (*see pp 287–288*). The beneficiaries under a will are not personally liable for IHT. Nor are the executors or the administrator (if there is no will), unless they distribute the estate while some IHT is still outstanding.

IHT always comes out of the deceased's estate, because it is a tax on the deceased's assets, not on anyone else. (Although there can be occasional scenarios where IHT is specifically attributable to a gift made during life and the recipient of the gift is liable for an IHT payment).

It is essential to note that payment of IHT must (usually) be made *before* the grant of probate. It must be made by the end of the sixth month after the month in which the deceased died (which can, therefore, be days more than six months, but always less than seven months). If not, HMRC will charge interest.[10] An IHT reference number must be obtained from HMRC (either online or by using form Schedule IHT422).

Banks and building societies can be asked to pay part or all of the IHT bill out of the deceased's account(s), if any. They will usually do so, paying direct to HMRC, using the Direct Payment Scheme (DPS), Form IHT423.

If there are just not enough funds available to pay IHT within the required six months, you can ask HMRC to **postpone payment** of some or all of the tax due until after probate is granted. This is called a 'grant on credit'. This would apply, for example, where the deceased owned a property but had very little money. Write to HMRC (with the heading: Grants on credit, plus the IHT reference number):

- request postponement
- tell HMRC how much tax you can pay now, and how much you can't
- explain why you can't (eg you cannot get release of bank funds or the sale of a property has not been completed)
- explain what steps will be taken to raise the funds to pay the tax
- send to HMRC, Inheritance Tax Team, BX9 1HT

If postponement is permitted, for example because of a property sale, you must pay **promptly** when the funds become available. The gov.uk web page, *Apply to postpone payment of Inheritance Tax* (April 2024), says, rather grumpily: 'If the tax is to be paid following the sale of a property, there must be an accepted offer and an estimated date for exchange of contracts. We cannot issue an open-ended undertaking without a clear date of when the tax will be paid.'

Alternatively, IHT may be paid, in relation to property (and, in one or two rare cases, certain specific assets) and with HMRC's agreement, by equal yearly instalments, up to ten years.[11] Use Form IHT400. This is an expensive option. HMRC will charge interest, currently at 7.5%, on the second and any further instalments. Payment by instalments could be made, for example, because it takes time to sell the deceased's house or because you (not a spouse or civil partner) inherit the house and wish to keep it to live in.

If the worst comes to the worst, and insufficient funds are available to pay the tax within the six months, the executor or administrator may need to obtain a temporary loan for the estate so that the estate can pay the tax on time – a loan from either personal funds or from a bank (and, of course, repayable from the estate in due course).

Once all the assets of the estate have been sold off, the executor (or administrator) must pay off any remaining outstanding IHT to HMRC.

If payment is late, HMRC may charge penalties and interest.

If there has been an overpayment to HMRC, for example a house has been sold for less than its estimated value as notified to HMRC, the balance to the estate (with interest) will be repaid by HMRC. If there has been an underpayment, because the property has been sold for more than the estimate, the increase could be declared on the estate tax return (*see pp 286–287*) as a capital gain; the tax on a capital gain is currently lower than IHT.

Further Guidance

Remember that this chapter is only a basic summary of the main provisions of IHT. Some guidance is provided at gov.uk, *How Inheritance Tax works: thresholds, rules and allowances* and at moneyhelper.org.uk, *A guide to Inheritance Tax*. MoneyHelper is a government-approved website, which provides independent and free guidance on money and pensions.

But if in doubt, seek expert advice from an IHT specialist.[12] This is not an easy subject.

Spouse or civil partner

If you have a long-term partner, there is an advantage in being married or in a civil partnership. Couples can pass their nil-rate band and residence nil-rate band IHT-free allowances on to their partner on death, but only if they are married or in a civil partnership (and UK domiciled).

Similarly, if married or in a civil partnership, but not otherwise, you can leave all your assets IHT free to your partner in your will. So, for example, if you are married with children, you and your spouse (or civil partner) could each make a will leaving your estate to your partner and on the partner's death to your children (or other 'direct descendants'[13]) equally (see p 16).

Under this kind of will, your spouse or civil partner pays no inheritance tax on your death, regardless of the size of the estate. On the surviving partner's death, the children will inherit equally, subject to IHT being paid. But the amount of IHT will be reduced as a result of the combined nil-rate bands and residence nil-rate bands from both partners, making a very substantial saving, not having to pay IHT on the first £1million of the estate (see also pp 130-131).

So if you have a partner but are not married or in a civil partnership, consider

- marriage or civil partnership, and then
- making a will leaving everything to your spouse or civil partner (and, after both deaths, to your children or other direct descendants)

To reduce the children's liability to pay IHT further, you could also consider making gifts to them during life, as above.

Tax Planning

IHT planning, if you choose to try and reduce the impact of inheritance tax on the beneficiaries of your estate, particularly children, is far from straightforward. I do not propose, for example, to go into deeds of variation or family trusts to offset liability for IHT. Life insurance policies may also be used to provide funds for beneficiaries so that they can pay IHT.

There are, however, a number of inheritance tax services which can reduce potential IHT. For example, there are investments in smaller businesses which qualify for some measure of business relief (BR), such as those on the Alternative Investment Market (AIM, ie not on a main stock exchange).[14] Some services require a two-year qualifying period (before death). Some ISAs, with investments up to £20,000 a year, and which hold assets qualifying for an IHT exemption, such as BR (above), can also be passed on in a will free of IHT.

These are complicated subjects. You need sound independent advice. Some of these services may be considered devices to avoid tax which you feel uncomfortable deploying. Some are investigated by HMRC from time to time. In 2019, for example, HMRC set up a unit to investigate the legality of 'family investment companies' (FICs), used by the better-off to reduce inheritance tax. However, HMRC concluded in 2021 that FICs were not indicative of tax avoidance or evasion.

As already discussed, gifts during life or charitable or political donations in a will are also ways of reducing IHT.

If you wish to begin with the basics of how to reduce your estate's liability for inheritance tax on your death, you would do well to consider the summary by the independent Office of Tax Simplification (OTS). The OTS lists for convenience the main exemptions, reliefs and thresholds as follows, all of which may reduce the IHT bill[15]:

Main exceptions, reliefs, thresholds

- Gifts to a spouse or civil partner
- Nil-rate band, transferable to spouse or civil partner: £325,000
- £3,000 annual gift exemption and £250 small gifts exemption
- Regular gifts from disposable income
- Residence nil-rate band for homes left to direct descendants, transferable to spouse or civil partner: £175,000
- Qualifying business or farm (subject to modification in 2026)
- Gifts to qualifying charities or political parties
- National heritage assets

What can you do about IHT?

1 Consider your property and other assets and decide whether to take expert independent advice about IHT planning (wealth succession)
2 Consider gifts during life or charitable bequests
3 Discuss inheritance with your children (or other beneficiaries) including a clear explanation of the details of your will
4 Consider reducing the value of your estate by spending money on a full and active retirement

Death and taxes and childbirth! There's never any convenient time for any of them.

Margaret Mitchell, *Gone with the Wind* (1936)

Future Changes to IHT?

There is much discussion about the pros and cons of IHT.

Some people are happy to let the state take a large portion of the value of their estate. It is money that will go to the general public purse and much-needed payment, for example, towards education and the NHS.

Some say that the tax falls mostly on the wealthy and is therefore appropriate taxation, redistributing wealth. If anything, it is argued, even though the higher UK income tax rates (at 40% and 45%) are some of the highest in the world, the scope of IHT should be enlarged, so as to tax the wealthy even more. An IHT charge results from the estate often including property. Any property that is transferred in life is taxable (capital gains tax and stamp duty), except between spouses, so why not on death?

Others argue that only a small number of estates are charged IHT. Under 5% of UK deaths each year lead to an IHT charge, a modest 27,800 deaths.[16] A better, clearer way of imposing a tax would be a property tax, based on a combination of the value of the property and the increase in value since purchase.

Others are less happy with IHT. They describe it as a 'toxic brand' which hits the middle classes hard. It is unfair because it taxes the super-rich and the less wealthy the same. And the rich are said to squirrel their money away more effectively anyway, particularly in trusts and AIM shares[17] which have some IHT exemption. It also motivates some to take their wealth out of the UK.

They also claim that IHT is double taxation, taxation already having been imposed on the money earned over a lifetime to create their estate and on the property which forms the greater part of the estate. And it is a tax which bites at the worst possible time, immediately after death. Others say that it is not double taxation because it is primarily a tax on property. That property is likely to have appreciated so substantially, by about 300% since 2000, that it is income which has not been taxed.

Some maintain that low IHT or no IHT at all would be a better incentive for working to provide for one's children and grandchildren and would reduce tax evasion schemes designed to avoid it, whereas others say that children and grandchildren should learn to make their own way in life.

On a more practical level, the rules of IHT, dating in their current form from 1986 (superseding Capital Transfer Tax), are considered to be complex and not easily understood. Even when no IHT is payable, a surviving spouse has to complete lengthy forms, which may involve the trouble and cost of professionals such as lawyers and estate agents. For the non-lawyer attempting to work out probate and IHT for themselves online, exemptions and reliefs are often seen to be unduly obscure.

Options for change

In 2018 the Government ordered a wide-ranging consultation about IHT. Chancellor Phillip Hammond said at the time that IHT was 'particularly complex' and asked for proposals to see if it was 'fit for purpose'.

Some of the varied suggestions for change made during this consultation included:

- A more aggressive form of the current IHT regime, targeting the wealthiest and reducing the extent of IHT exemptions such as extending the seven-year exemption for lifetime gifts to ten years.
- Taxing those who receive lifetime gifts (usually children or grandchildren) at a flat rate.
- Amending the thresholds, such as the nil-rate band, to keep pace with inflation. Or a flat-rate increase to, say, £500,000.
- Simplifying the different allowances and reliefs; providing simpler forms for easy online applications.
- Abolishing having to pay IHT to HMRC upfront before probate is granted.
- Abolishing IHT and taxing the capital gain in residential property at the time of transfer of title, during life or when enforced under a will after death.

The independent Office of Tax Simplification (OTS), which conducted the consultation, reported and made recommendations (July 2019). It found that there were many areas where Inheritance Tax was 'poorly understood, counter-intuitive, requires substantial record keeping ... or where the application of the law is simply unclear'. It made recommendations for change, retaining IHT, but amending and simplifying the process. None of these recommendations has yet been implemented.[18]

IHT is always reviewed by governments before every budget. Changes may be made at any time. Check gov.uk, MoneyHelper and other money websites for updates.

IHT remains in place

Two things, however, are certain.

First, IHT is not popular. Some call it the most hated tax, a 'death tax'. One opinion poll showed that 61% of those polled were against it, and that it was considered to be the most unfair of all taxes. The main reason given for this perception was that IHT represented 'double taxation' – just another tax, when taxes had already been paid on earnings and property purchase.[19] In practice the form-filling process is considered onerous and the whole process comes at a difficult time for grieving family members. Most people just do not know how it works. Some worry, incorrectly, that they will lose their home when their spouse dies.

Secondly, IHT is definitely a good little earner for the state. As stated above, it brings in over £7 billion a year,[20] with a rising number of estates affected.

Some economists see the next era as the 'non-inheritance' era. By this they mean that all the money the current younger generation might have inherited will be swallowed up by home care and care homes so that there will be nothing left to pass on. Others take a different view and see the younger generation as greater inheritors than the previous generation.

But, popular or not (and mostly not), IHT is likely to be here to stay, for some while anyway. Like it or not, those with estates which will be subject to an IHT charge, may like to think about it and what they can do about it.

Top Ten Tips

1	**Give thought to the totality of your estate:** property and other assets
2	**Make a will.** Consider leaving property and assets to your spouse or civil partner (to benefit from inherited nil-rate bands) (*see pp 128–130, 137–138*).
3	**Calculate the net value of your estate and how much IHT your estate is likely to be charged.** Take account of nil-rate bands (and inherited nil-rate bands).
4	**Consider whether you wish to let the state take IHT**, or whether you wish to try and reduce the IHT to be paid on your estate. Some people are happy for the state to take its share for the benefit of others.
5	**Consider making gifts to family** as some gifts during life are exempt from IHT
6	**Consider making gifts to charities** for tax relief
7	**Consider, if you want to, wider IHT planning.** Take expert advice and remember that you may need money in later life for care.
8	**Consider marriage or civil partnership if you're in a long-term relationship.** The IHT savings for your legal partner (on your death) are substantial.
9	**Discuss any IHT planning with close relatives.** It is better that they know in advance of your death.
10	**Look out for Government changes in IHT rules**; present figures are set for the foreseeable future but may change

CHAPTER 5

Scams

This chapter may cause some alarm. There may be plenty of frauds out there, some of them targeted at the elderly. But take heart. It is not your fault, and there is plenty you can do to keep fraudsters at bay. It is better to know about scams so as to be on guard as much as possible, rather than to ignore them.

Follow the steps below and you should be (mostly) fine.

How to Avoid Fraud

Before we look at individual types of fraud, there are a few basic steps which we should take at all times:

Dos:

- **Passwords** – Use strong passwords and different ones for bank accounts, financial organisations, credit cards, email accounts, etc.[1] Change passwords frequently. Use lower- and upper-case letters, numbers and punctuation.[2]
- **Security** – Install security software such as anti-virus for your computer. Set up two-factor authentication (2FA), sometimes called two-step verification, as an extra layer of security. Update software and apps frequently (updates will contain new security).
- **Screen lock** – Secure your smartphone and tablet with a screen lock (not your bank PIN).

- **Back up data** – Back up your most important data to an external hard drive or on a cloud-based storage system.
- **Bank accounts** – Check bank statements regularly (even daily) to look out for any unusual transactions. Notify the bank immediately of any.
- **Be aware** – Be on the lookout for the possibility of fraud, in phone calls or messages through text, email or on websites.
- **Double-check** – Check and double-check the possibility of fraud if you are in any doubt.

Don'ts:

- **Passwords** – Don't choose passwords which are easy to guess like Pa55word! or which use your name, family names, pet names or your date of birth.
- **Cold calls** – Do not respond to any cold calls out of the blue, particularly those which offer you attractive opportunities to make money, for example with pension funds (with offers of 'free pension review'). If an offer seems too good to be true, it probably is.
- **Pension pots** – Do not cash in pension pots without taking sound independent and regulated financial advice.
- **Door-to-door** – Don't buy goods or services (such as roofing, tiling or driveway repairs) from a seller who turns up out of the blue (unless you are sure about them). Don't let a stranger into your house on an excuse (unless you are sure about them).
- **Bank details** – Do not give bank details or any personal details which might lead to fraudsters getting into your accounts out over the phone. (Unless *you* make the call to a guaranteed secure number – even then be cautious).
- **Payments** – Do not make a substantial payment to a bank account until you have double-checked with the payee (*see below*).
- **Links in emails** – Don't respond to any unexpected and unusual emails. In particular, do not click on a link in the email: it may infect your computer with a virus and gain access to personal and banking details.

Different Types of Fraud

LOOK OUT for these scams

1. Cold calling
2. Phone fraud
3. Door-to-door
4. Identity fraud
5. Phishing
6. Fake websites
7. Pension, investment fraud
8. Authorised push payments
9. Advance fee payments
10. Romance fraud

Frauds keep changing with the times (as do their names), such as scams in a pandemic or an energy crisis or a war. *Action Fraud*, below, lists over 160 different types of fraud.[3] We all need to be on the lookout, not just for ourselves but for others we care for who may be vulnerable.

Fraud is now the most prevalent crime in the UK, over 40% of all crime.[4] Losing money to a fraudster, and usually these days that means an invisible fraudster, is a very distressing experience. We are all capable of being exploited at a moment of weakness (or even, dare I say, at a moment of greed).

The following ten types of fraud are, sadly, common enough. Some overlap. We are all likely to come across one or more, particularly in this digital age. But if you keep a watchful eye out and follow the tips, you will minimise the risk of loss.

1. Cold calling

If someone calls you out of the blue trying to sell you something, in a phone call you are not expecting, stop the call, particularly if they want to interest you in any of the following:

- pensions advice
- investment in the stock market or bonds
- the purchase of land or parcels of land or forestry or property overseas
- renewable energy schemes
- just about anything that will make you money, lots of money

They will promise high interest rates, exotic returns, quick rewards, adventurous schemes. They will be charming, persuasive, apparently helpful, and sound perfectly normal. But they are fraudsters. They don't care about you. They are targeting you because you are an older person and there is a chance you will be susceptible to their wiles. Not pretty, but true.

Cold callers who make promises of financial gains should be avoided at all costs. They are probably a scam. Cold calling often relates to pension funds because of the relaxation of rules about pension pots since 2015 (*see below and pp 163–166*).

Cold calling on the phone is sufficiently common for BT to have advised customers that it is 'probably a scam if someone calls you out of the blue' to:

- tell you that your service has been hacked
- tell you they've found a problem with your computer
- try remotely to take control of your computer or another device
- ask you for an urgent payment and threaten to disconnect your service
- ask for payment details to activate any of BT's landline features, such as BT Call Protect or Caller Display

For malicious or fraudulent calls, BT has a Nuisance Calls Advice Line on 0800 661 441.[5]

The message is clear: if in doubt, cut the call off. Or ask the caller to put it in writing.

'Family' text or WhatsApp message.

A cold caller by text or WhatsApp may falsely pretend to be a family member – 'Hi Mum' – who needs help as they have lost their phone or their phone is damaged and a bill needs paying urgently.

In 2023, the Government announced an intention to extend the ban on cold calling in relation to pensions to cold calling about consumer financial services and products.[6]

WHAT TO DO?

- If someone calls unexpectedly and tries to sell you something, stop the call
- Never share your personal or bank details with such a caller
- Do not cash in your pension pots without receiving professional, independent FCA-approved financial advice.
- If in doubt, check and double check

2. Phone fraud

Fraudsters sometimes pose as banks, utility companies or government agencies, in fact any institution you would be likely to trust, such as the NHS (in Covid times), HMRC, Citizens Advice, even the police. They may call up and ask you to move money from your bank account into a new one. No bank would ever do that, not on the phone (nor in texts or emails). But the fraudsters may have acquired some information about you in advance which makes them sound more plausible. Do not respond.

If in doubt, **check with your bank** (or other institution). Use the fraud phone number on the back of your bank card. Keeping a list of genuine numbers to hand is also helpful. One of the best ways to protect yourself is to **check your bank transactions regularly** (weekly, even daily) to check for anything unusual. If in doubt, contact your bank straightaway.

Banks and other institutions give out warning messages repeatedly:

- **Never give out personal and banking details on the phone** (or by email or text), unless you are absolutely sure you are speaking to your bank (or other institution). Just a few personal details may be enough for a fraudster to persuade a bank they are genuine (when they are not). Even a full name or date of birth may be enough for a fraudster to bypass security.
- **Never give out a PIN or password on the phone** (or by email or text).
- **Never transfer money out of your account following a phone request** (for example when the caller has said your account is at risk of fraud and demanded urgent action)
- **Never agree to help with an internal investigation**
- **Never agree to hand over cash or a card to a courier**

Some disguised deceits counterfeit truth so perfectly that not to be taken in by them would be an error of judgment.

La Rochefoucauld, *Maxims* (1665)

The fraudsters may give a persuasive reason such as 'Your account is no longer secure because fraudsters have hacked into it'. In one example, a real case, a gang posing as police officers persuaded a number of older people, some in their eighties and nineties, to take cash out of their accounts and hand it over to couriers who came to collect it. This gang was caught, but that is often not the case. Older people had 'helped' the 'police' because they trusted them. But some of the victims felt foolish afterwards and suffered a loss of confidence: 'I felt such an idiot.' Some lost much-needed life savings.

Older people may be more vulnerable to this kind of scam because they have been loyal customers of the same bank, often for decades. A call from somebody pretending to be from that bank is likely to sound more plausible. This is sometimes called 'number spoofing'.

We all have to be on the lookout. For ourselves and for those we look after. Data suggests that bank scams have been substantial in recent years, with losses of over £700 million a year.[7]

Sometimes a team of fraudsters will operate using the same pre-prepared script. Apps to identify this are being developed now. It is hoped that they will be able to recognise repeated patterns of words and phrases and warn the intended victim to look out and double-check.

False urgency is a common feature of some of these fraudulent phone calls, telling the victim there is something they have to deal with straightaway. This may be particularly confusing for some older people. Ignore any conversation beginning with 'I am calling from HMRC to discuss very recent fraudulent activity we have discovered on your account' or 'I am calling from the City of London Police Fraud Department because your bank account has been hacked into', and anything that includes the words 'This requires immediate action by you' is also probably fake.

Urgent action may be encouraged on the phone (or in fraudulent email or text messages) telling you that your TV licence or some other service is about to expire and that payment is needed 'right now'. Spam emails frequently use phrases such as 'Last Reminder', 'Last Warning', 'Final Notice'. Beware. Sometimes threats are made, too, such as 'Unless you act now your account will be closed down in three hours' or 'I am calling from the criminal court in Birmingham; an arrest warrant will be issued unless you pay this tax bill.'

There is also SIM-swap fraud, where a fraudster manages to hack into your phone and make banking transactions without your knowledge or permission. They might, for example, be payments to well-known insurance companies. The fraudster uses names so you don't at first worry about the payment, even if you see it on your bank statements. But if it works once or twice the modest payments will increase in amount and frequency. There is nothing you can do about this except **check your bank**

accounts regularly. If you see any unusual transaction, contact the bank immediately.

Fraudsters may also hack into your phone and copy genuine texts from your bank and then slip in a text to you which looks just like a text from your bank and says something like: 'Have you just made a purchase of £400, if not please call on the following number'. You think it is genuine and call the bank, aka the fraudsters, and provide information over the phone about your bank account.

This can all be rather confusing in this digital age. Although there is more protection from data loss than ever before, there is also a constant barrage of demands from legitimate companies for personal details.

Banking online (on a computer) or using a banking app (on a smartphone) gives you immediate access to your account(s). This way you can check your account(s) regularly. If anything is out of place you can phone the bank on the right number. Most of you will, I am sure, know what an app is and how to use one. But in case you don't, I have spelt it out.*

** **What is an app?** An app is a software 'application' or computer programme. It is most commonly used as a mobile app, for a smartphone* or tablet. An app helps you perform certain functions and may store data. For example, a banking app lets you access your bank accounts, make transfers and payments, and check details that are stored. A game app gives you a game to play. Other apps will help you order food or a cab. Some are free. Some you pay for.*

** **What is a smartphone?** A smartphone is a mobile phone plus. It is not just a phone, making and receiving calls (like a landline phone). It is also a computer with computer functions like access to the internet and apps (above).*

Take action. If you have been conned and then realise it, you should **tell your bank (the genuine bank) immediately**.

Or call 159 (preferably on another phone) to Stop Scams UK which will connect you safely and directly to your bank.

WHAT TO DO?

- **Beware of companies/organisations calling you out of the blue unexpectedly**
- If in doubt when on the phone, you can always ask them to put their request in writing
- Never share your personal or bank details with an unexpected caller
- Make sure any payment you make goes to the correct person or organisation; ask for confirmation it has been safely received
- Check the details of your bank accounts regularly (every day, if possible)
- Always have your bank's fraud helpline number to hand
- If you discover your phone has been hacked, make sure the SIM card is changed

3. Door-to-Door

Beware door-to-door sellers. A kindly face may knock on your door out of the blue and suggest that your roof needs some re-tiling (particularly after a storm) or your chimney stack needs repointing or your drive needs doing up. You didn't know you needed this work, but you agree to the work being done, a deposit is taken and you never see them again. Worse still, they start the work, take money, then say the job is worse than they thought and take more money, then disappear with a botched job or a job

We are inclined to believe those whom we do not know because they have never deceived us.

Dr Johnson, *The Idler* (1758)

hardly done at all. Or even worse, the demands for more money are backed up by threats.

There may, of course, always be genuine callers at the front door, such as charity workers, campaigners and political canvassers. But **if somebody calls at your door out of the blue, offering to sell you something (whether goods or services) and you haven't ordered it, be wary**. You probably won't need it, whatever it is, and even if you do need it, that's not the way to go about it. If it's building work, for example, get the job done properly. Get comparative quotes. Find builders who are recommended by people you can trust.

Be careful of fraudsters who turn up unannounced and pretend to be somebody official, like a Trading Standards Officer, suggesting that money is owed and demanding immediate payment. Or they may offer help with loft insulation if you pay into a 'green deal' grant scheme. Genuine green-deal energy-saving schemes may be available, but they won't be offered to you on the doorstep.

Banks are supposed to keep an eye on unusual transactions by elderly customers, through the Banking Protocol.[8] This encourages bank staff to call the police urgently when they are suspicious, for example about an older customer taking out a large sum of cash.

There is another knock on the door. This time a dishevelled young man apologises and says: 'Could I just have a drink of water?' Being a generous soul you let him in and before you know it he has taken cash and cards from your handbag or petty cash float, even the car key, and disappeared with a cheery wave or possibly no wave at all. Or it might be a recce for a burglary.

There is yet another knock on the door. (You are having a bad day.) It is late in the evening and the caller, charming and friendly as ever, apologises and says that they need to get to the hospital urgently because their mother has been in an accident and they've come out without any money. So could they borrow some? Or they need cash to get a cab home because they've missed the last bus and have no cash. Or some other sob story.

There are plenty of variations on this. And they may even offer to leave their watch or phone as security, promising to bring the money back tomorrow. The amount will only be small. But the fraudster, who of course never cares about his victim, will repeat this to numerous houses, preying on people's generosity and kindness. I turned one away once (and I have had more than one at the door) and saw him rushing down the street going from house to house, quickly though, in case anyone called the police.

WHAT TO DO?

- Don't let any stranger into your house unless they have an appointment
- If you let anyone in, they should be watched and your small item valuables should have been put safely away
- Don't agree to have repair work done by a stranger who knocks on your door; if work needs doing get it from a builder recommended by a trustworthy friend
- If you decide to give money to strangers (it's your choice), the amount should be modest

4. Identity fraud

Identity fraud is when personal details are stolen and used to commit fraud.

All the fraudster needs are a few personal details about you and your bank. They then open an account or buy something in your name without your knowledge or permission. And off they go.

Identity fraud raises its ugly head in a number of ways, for example in phone fraud (above). Identity fraud counts for more than half of all fraud (with nearly all of it online), according to Cifas, the UK fraud prevention service. The over-sixties are targeted more than any other age group.[9]

Do not give out your personal or banking details to anyone without checking first. This is a must. Organisations, like banks, already have your details. Except for limited security clearance details, they won't ask for them over the phone or online. If it's a bank, you can always go into your local bank (if you have one) and explain, taking ID with you. They won't mind your sensible caution.

The Dedicated Card and Payment Crime Unit (DCPCU) advises that every request for personal or financial details or to transfer money should be checked and double checked – every time.

You should **check your credit card and bank accounts as often as possible**, daily if you can. It is easier to do that if you have a banking app on a smartphone. Checking regularly means that if you see a transaction you don't recognise you can report it quickly to your bank. If you do, you are more likely to get your money back from the bank.

Update your mobile phone, computer or tablet when asked to; that increases security. Consider internet security software.

Online banking has grown fast, and fraud has grown with it too. But although 90% of people aged 25–34 use online banking, that percentage drops to 51% for those aged 65–74, to 38% for those aged 75–79 and to 18% for those aged 80 plus.[10]

WHAT TO DO?

- If you need to provide your bank details (name and number of account, sort code) by email or text in order to receive money by bank transfer, make sure you know exactly who is getting them
- Shred your personal details and bank details on paper documents rather than throwing them out
- Change your passwords regularly and always make them difficult to guess

5. Phishing

Phishing is a **false email** pretending to come from a reputable company or organisation such as a bank or TV Licensing or HMRC or BT. It is an impersonation scam.

The email is designed to obtain personal details such as usernames, passwords, credit card details, PIN numbers[11] and bank account details. These emails look authentic but they are false. Do not respond to them. Do not click on links. Delete them.

The same applies with phishing by **text**, sometimes called SMS phishing or smishing. WhatsApp groups may also be targeted, usually by a fraudster claiming to be a genuine member of the group.

With a little information about you, fraudsters may be able to persuade a bank that they can pass security – on your account. Or they may be able to access funds or further information with a username and password. So they fish for it. It is known as 'phishing'.[12]

Fraudsters may also **phone** you pretending to be a reputable company or organisation.

What tricks do the scammers use?

- They may call you a valued customer.
- They may say that fraud has been suspected on your bank account and you need to confirm certain details. Don't.
- They may say that an attempt has been made to withdraw money from your account from overseas. Can you confirm certain details? Don't.
- You may be asked to go to a website link and provide information. Don't. Don't click on the link. It may lead to hacking into your email account. Don't provide information at all. It could be used against you. That is the fraudster's intention.
- They pretend to be from TV Licensing and ask you to set up a new direct debit: 'Something's gone wrong with your payments'.
- They pretend to be from HMRC. 'You are entitled to a tax rebate' or 'tax refund'. (HMRC themselves invite you to report suspicious emails to the genuine email address phishing@hmrc.gov.uk or to forward suspicious texts to the genuine text number 60599.)
- They pretend to be from a delivery company requiring further details to make the delivery.
- **False urgency**. The scam contains a threat (urgent action must be taken or else) or a reward such as a refund, rebate, overpayment to be returned; eg inviting you to claim for an energy bill rebate, by registering your bank details.

- If you click on the link, as requested, you will be asked to provide further details; you may then get a phone call from your 'bank' (the fraudster), requesting you to transfer money to a 'safe account' (the fraudster's account).

A TV Licensing scam email sent to me was as follows:

Email subject heading

#Something's gone wrong with your payments#] | Review Automated Confirmation 'We are sorry to let you know that the TV License could not be automatically renewed' | Automated renew on 11/23/2022 12:55:02 a.m. #

Text of email

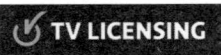

You are covered until 11/23/2022 12:55:02 a.m.

Dear [my email address] TV Licensing Customer,

This is an automatic email sent by TV Licensing Customer Service system. Please do not reply to this email, as any messages sent to this address will not receive a response.

We are sorry to let you know that the TV License could not be automatically renewed. Something's gone wrong with your payments

As we couldn't take the latest payment from your bank account, this amount will also need to be paid when you set up your new Direct Debit.

[LINK to bogus website: **Setup New Direct Debit** etc]

Remember, if you don't keep up with your payments, we may be forced to cancel your license or pass your details to a debt collection agency.

Thanks

TV Licensing

Important Notice: The content of this email is intended only for use by the individual or entity to whom it is addressed. If you have received this email by mistake, please advise the sender and delete the message and attachments immediately. This email, including attachments, may contain confidential, sensitive, legally privileged and/or copyright information.

How to (try and) spot a fraudulent email

There are a number of points to note about the fraudulent email (above) which was not from the real TV Licensing (although used their real logo):

- The sender's email address (which I have not copied) was not the official TV Licensing website, although it looked official. TV Licensing usually only use donotreply@tvlicensing.co.uk or donotreply@spp.tvlicensing.co.uk.
- Next to it on the right and **in faint letters, under the downward arrow**, was an apparently private email address ending in @telenet.be (a Belgian email address).
- The email is directed to me in an email address name with the words 'TV Licensing Customer'. Most scams use a generic title like this or address you as 'Dear Customer' without using your name. Genuine companies or organisations will usually address you by name.
- The subject heading of the email was: 'Something's gone wrong with your payments'. This is a familiar scam. So is 'You are due a refund because you have overpaid.'
- The link website was a scam. If I had clicked on it I would have been asked to set up a Direct Debit for a fraudulent account. A good tip[13]: **Do not click on the link, but let your mouse (or finger on laptop) hover over the link**. It will show you the name of the website underneath. In my case it was old.bigom.com etc, which does not exactly look like the genuine TV Licensing website.
- False emails often have written mistakes in the text. Poor spelling, grammar or punctuation. In the above email there are two slight punctuation mistakes.
- The date in numbers was unusual, using the American style with the month before the day.

Another example of phishing fraud, this time a text message:

> **Text Message**
> Today 17:52
>
> GOVUK: Your are eligible for a discounted energy bill under the Energy Bills Support Scheme. You can apply here: https://mysupport-scheme.com

If you receive a fake email or text like either of these, delete them. Never click on the link. Never provide any personal details. If you are asked to phone a number, do not, unless you are absolutely sure it is genuine.

Phishing comes in all sorts of guises. There is spear phishing, directed at specific individuals or companies, or bulk phishing which targets more randomly. Usually there will be a link in the message. Avoid the link. Do not click on it.

Voice phishing involves a call purporting to come from a genuine bank or other trusted organisation. It invites you to call the bank on a number and then asks basic security questions. Do not call the bank on that number. Do not answer security questions unless you are absolutely sure you are on the line to your genuine bank. Do not ask a (fraudulent) caller for a bank number to check the authenticity of the call. Only call your bank on a trusted number you have separately. Check the call via an independently reliable source. If in doubt, check and double check.

HMRC report that a common bogus phone call in their name claims: 'HMRC is filing a lawsuit against you ...' If true, you would get a letter through the post.

Another example of voice phishing: fraudsters have posed over the phone as officers of the National Crime Agency (NCA), specifically targeting older people.[14] They claim that your phone has been hacked into by criminals and that you 'must move your money to a safe account'. Do not move your money to their account.

When this first came to light, the NCA put this specific warning on its website:

An NCA officer will NEVER:
✗ Ask for remote access to your computer
✗ Ask you to verify your personal details, such as passwords, account numbers or card details via phone, email or online
✗ Ask you to transfer or hand over money via phone, email or online or on the doorstep
✗ Speak or act in a threatening manner

Take action. If you have been innocently caught out, and provided details for example about your bank, **contact your bank** on the fraudline or other genuine number (or in any quick legitimate way) **immediately**. We all make mistakes.

WHAT TO DO?

- Check unexpected emails or texts from organisations you would normally trust - are they genuine on this occasion?
- Only use the bank's dedicated website or genuine phone inquiry number on bank cards to provide information to your bank
- DON'T CLICK ON LINKS – hover the cursor over the link (without clicking on it) to see and check the website underneath – it may provide access to your email account if you click

SCAMS

> *** What is a URL?** A URL (Uniform Resource Locator) is an internet web address. For example, the genuine URL for TV Licensing is https://www.tvlicensing.co.uk.

6. Fake websites

Always use official websites. If you need a government website for a specific form, check for the correct site. If you make an internet search, listings at the top of the page are often paid for by private companies. Look instead for the gov.uk website.

Copycat websites pretend to be official websites when they are not. They will try and sell you an official document when it is free. For example, charging the over-seventies for a driving licence when it can be renewed for free on the genuine DVLA website. Or charging for HMRC tax forms when they are free or passport applications in excess of the real fee.

For official stuff you want the gov.uk website address. For security, join the Government Gateway ID service. It is free and you will choose your own password.

Check whether an official document or permit is free or, if not, what the official price is. Some websites will offer a 'special speedy' service for a permit, but at an inflated price, and it won't be any quicker.

Ticket fraud – Be careful when you buy a ticket for a concert, sporting event or other event. Over £6.5 million is lost from fake tickets or non-existent tickets every year.[15]

Look out for bogus websites, particularly those which have a URL (an internet web address) which is similar to the real one but different. This sort of thing happens when there is a big sporting event coming up such as the football World Cup. If the sporting event is in the USA, for example, there will be false websites offering Esta permits, USA visas. Look out for fake tickets when very popular rock and pop concerts sell out quickly. To be on the safe side, only buy from clearly authorised websites, the promoter, official agents or reputable ticket exchange sites. Pay by credit card not bank transfer.

There may be a lottery scam too, such as 'You have won the FIFA lottery, please send details to claim your winnings.'

Holiday accommodation is a kind of fraud that is said to be on the increase. Scammers set up bogus websites offering holiday accommodation that does not exist or use genuine websites to list genuine properties that are not available to rent. Attractive looking websites may display offers with special discounts. Beware. Check and double check.

Charity websites, even those using real logos such as Save the Children, may be fake. Hundreds of fakes sprang up to encourage donations to support people or troops in Ukraine. Check carefully. Your money is needed, but in the right place.

If you come across any fake site, it helps if you report it. Report to Action Fraud (online or 0300 123 2040) and/or to the National Trading Standards eCrime Team.

WHAT TO DO?

- If you want an official document, such as an application form or a permit, **use only the gov.uk website**
- If a website makes a charge, check whether it should be free
- For online purchases, check and double check that the website is genuine

7. Pension fraud; investment fraud

Pension fraud has risen dramatically since 2015, following the relaxation of pension fund rules. Chancellor George Osborne decided to give those who are 55 and over the chance to access their previously tied-up pension funds and convert them (or part of them) into cash (*see pp 121–122*).

Fraudsters realised that some pensioners, with access to pension funds, might be easy targets. If they could be attracted by promises of riches, they might take their money out of existing and genuine pension schemes and 'invest' it in fraudulent pension or other investment schemes. Schemes showing pictures of luxury goods and expensive cars appeared online. In some cases an impressive-sounding 'free' review of your pension and other funds was offered. Their aim? To get you to invest in 'exciting' investment schemes which don't exist. They get their hands on your money. You get nothing.

Pension scammers are the lowest of the low. They rob savers of their hard-earned retirement and devastate lives.

John Glen MP, Economic Secretary to the Treasury (January 2019)

There is an increasing number of seemingly attractive offers on Facebook and Instagram (Meta), sometimes 'endorsed' by photos of celebrities. Many scams offer mouth-watering returns from shares, bonds, foreign exchange and cryptocurrencies (cryptoassets). They come from firms not authorised by the Financial Conduct Authority (FCA).

Surprisingly, research suggests that pension holders are nine times more likely to accept 'advice' (and make an impulse buy) from someone online than they would from a stranger face to face.

Please DO

- Be wary of any cold call out of the blue, however attractive it may sound
- Consider carefully whether it is genuine or too good to be true
- Take independent financial advice before investing
- Check the Financial Conduct Authority's ScamSmart website page to check a pension or investment opportunity you've been offered: fca.org.uk/scamsmart

Please DON'T

- Be tempted to take the bait
- Listen or talk
- Provide financial information or banking details
- **Hand over money**

Pension scams are said to cost savers as much as £5 million per year even though since 2019 scammers have faced fines of up to £500,000. Losses through pension scams can be huge. The average loss per person is said to be £75,000, although lower average figures have also been reported.[16]

Cold-calling about pensions and pension products was banned in 2019. Online scams involving 'binary options' trading are popular despite also being banned.[17] They are little more than high-risk betting on a financial index, whether it will go up or down.[18] A man from Bournemouth was sentenced to seven years' imprisonment for defrauding 300 investors, many of them friends and employees, out of £22 million. They invested in his 'lucrative' futures trading fund, SureInvestment. All they invested in was his lavish lifestyle. Charm and good salesmanship are often hallmarks of the successful fraudster.

It seems that plenty of us may be tempted. A report by the Financial Conduct Authority (FCA) and the Pensions Regulator has suggested that nearly 25% of those aged 55 and over would be tempted to respond to an interesting sounding offer from a cold caller on pension plans.[19] As one pension firm put it, pension pots are 'a juicy target'[20] (*see p 148*).

Billions have been taken out by those over 55 since the change in the law in 2015. The average withdrawal in recent times has been over £7,000, even though they may be hit by taxation. In 2021–22 access to pension pots increased by 22% to £45,638 million, but fell in 2022–23 to £43,199 million.[21]

If you are tempted to take money out of your pension pot to try and beat the annuity rate:

- Take proper independent financial advice from an approved independent financial adviser (IFA); check that the IFA is registered with the Financial Conduct

Authority (FCA): see the Financial Services Register at register.fca.org.uk
- Preferably deal only with a reputable company that has been recommended to you by someone you can absolutely trust
- Check scam investments on the FCA Warning List at fca.org.uk, *Be a ScamSmart investor*
- Never respond to cold callers (above)
- Consider: if promised investment returns sound too good to be true, they probably are
- Be wary that dealing with genuine investment companies may not guarantee that your annuity can be beaten; and watch out for high charges

Land banking schemes are a variation of investment frauds. You are offered a plot of land which will 'increase substantially in value once planning permission is granted'. If the land exists, which it may not, permission is rarely granted and the purchase is more or less worthless.

If you are the slightest bit interested in such a scheme, check that the company or individual is FCA registered and approved. The FCA also has a warning list of firms to avoid.

WHAT TO DO?

- Do not respond to cold callers offering pension advice or attractive investment opportunities (such as land or crypto currency deals)
- If you wish to take out cash from your pension funds, take advice from a proper independent financial adviser (IFA) who is listed with the FCA
- If you choose to take from your pension fund and re-invest, check the cost of the re-investment charges; only re-invest with a reputable, tried and trusted company
- Don't part with any substantial sum without checking and double checking authenticity

8. Authorised push payments

Be careful whenever you make a substantial payment.

'Authorised push payments' (APP frauds) are a common fraud, mostly originating online. There are over 230,000 cases reported and gross annual losses of nearly £460 million.[22]

In this fraud, **a bank customer is tricked into sending money to an account outside their control**. For example, the fraudster poses as a genuine person, such as the victim's solicitor or builder, and deceives the victim into making a payment into a fraudulent account. Often the fraudster will hack into the solicitor or builder's genuine email account and intercept or divert a payment.

To give a real example, the victim employed a solicitor to help them purchase a house. The solicitor was in regular email contact with the house buyer (victim). At the point when a deposit for the purchase was due, the fraudster hacked into the solicitor's account and sent an email in the name of the solicitor to the victim with details of a bank account. Without double-checking with the solicitor, the victim paid the deposit into the fraudster's account and the money was gone. This is sometimes known as 'malicious redirection'.

In another real-life example, a house owner was having extensive building works done at home. They had been in regular email contact with the builder. There had been a dispute between them about some additional payments and at the point when this was nearly resolved, the fraudster hacked into the builder's email account and requested the final payment into a particular account (the fraudster's account). Without double-checking, the victim paid the bill and several thousand pounds were lost.

There have been variations of APP fraud, usually involving payments online or through social media. They could involve, for example, making a payment or part payment in advance for a product or service, such as a car, TV or holiday rental, which may never have existed (known as 'malicious payee'). Fraudsters sometimes pretend to be 'bank security staff' and demand that money is moved immediately for safe-keeping to another account, which is in fact the fraudster's account.

Reimbursement

This has been something of a controversial topic. Recovering the loss, which may be considerable, may not be so easy. Banks have in some cases shown a reluctance to compensate for APP fraud, arguing that the victim has not done enough to protect the payment. In some cases they have refused reimbursement because the victim is said to have been 'grossly negligent' or just 'careless', even though the fraud has clearly been sophisticated and the elderly targeted. In 2022, the reimbursement figure only reached just over 50% for the first time.[23] Some banks are better at recompense than others. For example, in 2023 TSB refunded 88% of total losses, whereas Monzo refunded only 17%.[24]

Most banks have clear **warnings** on screen for substantial payments, with drop-down boxes, questions, etc. **It is up to you to be very careful. To check and double-check, before and after any substantial payment.**

On the other hand, some banks have been slow to match names with account details, despite the fact that a payment to a bank should and does require a payee's name to be entered by the victim. A 'Confirmation of Payee' system, with a regulatory direction to the banks on matching, was introduced in 2020 (updated in 2022), although it still places the onus on the customer to get the payment right.[25]

A voluntary Contingent Reimbursement Model (CRM) Code,[26] was in place for reimbursement by banks from 2019. Santander, for example, signed up to the Code in early 2020, but straightaway warned its customers:

Please note that we will not refund you if we find that you should have known that you were sending money to a fraudster – although we will always take circumstances into consideration.

In October 2024 the scheme became mandatory.[27] Victims of APP scams, often involving substantial sums of money, must be compensated (with the sending and receiving bank splitting the loss 50:50) and, in most cases, within five days, so long as the claim is made by the customer within 13 months of the fraud.

But there are **limitations**. Reimbursement is capped at £85,000 per scam. This figure, which has been reduced from £415,000 (and which falls in line with the customer protection limit for bank accounts), means that some victims will not be compensated in full, however sophisticated the fraud which has duped them.

There are other exceptions (escape clauses for banks?) which may restrict recompense. If the bank can show that the customer acted with **'gross negligence'**, no obligation to reimburse arises. What does 'gross negligence' mean in this context? It is difficult to tell. What's more, even though the onus is upon the bank to show that there has been gross negligence, it will be the bank who will decide whether there has been gross negligence. This could therefore favour the bank, allowing it to argue in some cases that the customer is at fault and should not be reimbursed.[28]

On the other hand, if the customer is **'vulnerable'** (also yet to be decided what that means precisely, but may include some older persons), the bank will have to reimburse the customer automatically, without considering whether the customer had acted with gross negligence.[29]

If the bank fails to reimburse you, go to the Financial Ombudsman Service (FOS) for help: *see pp 95-96*. They deal with thousands of complaints about frauds and scams, the most common being APP fraud. The FOS may, in some cases, be able to secure compensation which exceeds the PSR limit of £85,000. Their website tells you how to complain.[30]

WHAT TO DO?

- Check and double check any substantial payment **before** and **after** making it:
  - **Before:** confirm the payment details using at least two independent methods, for example looking up a telephone number (eg on a professional register) and calling it to verify details given in an email or letter
  - **After:** confirm that your payment has been received safely that day and ask for an immediate receipt
- If the payment is to a solicitor, for example, check **before** with the genuine solicitor that all details, particularly bank account details, are correct, and check with the solicitor immediately **after** payment that the payment has been received
- Keep a written record of all the dealings of each transaction
- If you have any doubt about the payment, check with your bank
- If your bank refuses to reimburse you for a scam, put your complaint in writing and then, if you make no progress, complain to the Financial Ombudsman

9. Advance fee payments

This type of fraud involves tricking the victim into paying money up front in order to 'unlock' funds which have, for example, been 'won' or 'inherited'.

Lottery fraud. You are informed you have won a lottery prize (which does not exist). You are asked to send money in order to release the 'winnings' (which you will never see).

Inheritance fraud. Similarly, you are informed that a long-lost relative has died in a far-off country and has left you an 'inheritance' (which does not exist). You are asked to send money to release the funds or to send bank or credit card details so that the funds (which you will never receive) can be sent to you.

WHAT TO DO?

- As always, beware the unexpected and check carefully
- Don't pay for anything in advance without tangible, verifiable evidence that it will be delivered later

10. Romance fraud

Lonely-hearts and dating websites are popular. But there are fraudsters out there (mostly online and **often invisible**) trying to take older people for a ride, particularly those in the 65–74 age bracket. Some older people may be vulnerable because they are lonely and more willing to be trusting than they should be.[31] Romance fraud is on the increase. It is in the top five of types of reported frauds. Annual losses from this type of fraud total more than £92 million. The average loss per person is £11,500, with an average of ten payments per case.[32]

The fraudster will try and develop a 'loving, caring' relationship with the older person, showing a 'kind and compassionate' nature. And, if online, being or pretending to be a person of a similar age, often with a fake profile and a fake picture. Fraudsters often appear charming and trustworthy. But they are manipulative and sometimes coercive. They will work on building up a level of trust, praising and complimenting you.

Then they will ask for money, maybe just a loan (which will never be repaid), or outright cash, often for highly emotive, personal reasons, intended to tug at the heart strings. The money may be for 'medical costs after an accident', because of 'the need to fund special cancer treatment only available in the USA', to help fund 'special care' for a child, or to help fund 'a deposit for a dependent child to buy a house'. The money may be for a 'cannot fail investment' or to support a business which will be 'bound to succeed'. They will nearly always be false.

CrimeStoppers suggests one or two tell-tale signs[33]:

- the relationship is progressed by the fraudster with **undue haste**
- the fraudster tries to take the conversation off the website or social media platform on to a more private platform, such as WhatsApp
- the fraudster makes excuses why they can't meet up or why they can't video chat
- the fraudster claims to be working overseas in the military or medical profession
- when the fraudster asks for money it's **urgent**, for an emergency, they try to rush you
- the fraudster tells you to keep your relationship private and not tell anyone

If you are a kind and generous person, think twice before lending or giving money to your 'new friend' (or of making a financial transaction on their behalf). Can you afford to lose the money? How much money is it? It may start small and then get bigger. Talk to someone you trust for advice.

WHAT TO DO?

- Be wary of someone not prepared to speak on camera or face-to-face
- **Don't lend or give money to someone you have never or only recently met**
- If you are tempted to help them, double check if you can, eg checking when the money is said to be for medical care
- **Confide in a trusted relative or friend** before making important decisions about money or property with a 'new friend', so that you can discuss any request for money openly

What Do You Do When You Think You May Be a Victim?

Keep a record. As soon as you suspect fraud, make a written record of all transactions, conversations and communications, with dates and times, and names if known. This will be invaluable in the process of claiming redress.

Take advice. If you need advice, contact your local Citizens Advice, call 0808 223 1133.

Report to the bank. Report any loss or unusual activity to your bank immediately. Do not delay. Report suspected fraud to the bank's fraud number. Or call 159 to Stop Scams UK which will connect you safely and directly to your bank.

Monitor your bank accounts regularly (every day if possible). Smartphone apps and online banking make this easy. Look out for unusual activity. Check unusual payments, for example payments to insurance companies that on the face of it look legitimate and may not at first blush look like a scam.

Keep a record of any calls, emails or other contact with your bank. Keep a record of the dates, times and content. You may need to look back over the details if there is a dispute over reimbursement.

Report to police. If you believe you are the victim of crime, you should always report the offence to the police. Do not delay. Keep a record of your report.

You should report the crime to the police and to *Action Fraud* (*below*).

In some cases the police may give you **a crime reference number**. But in most cases you will be referred to Action Fraud. If the police have not already, Action Fraud will give you a police crime reference number when you report to them. The bank or insurance company may require it.

If you have been defrauded and the bank has paid you back, you may be reluctant to report to the police. That is up to you. But if there is any uncertainty about recompense by the bank, you should report to the police. The bank may take you more seriously if you do.

Do not necessarily expect a speedy response. One think tank has estimated that for each police worker dedicated to economic crime, there are 2,500 fraud crimes each year.[34]

Report to Action Fraud[35], the UK's national reporting centre for fraud and cybercrime (any computer-oriented crime) since 2009, used by all police forces since 2012.[36] The UK government, however, announced that it would be replaced by an as-yet-unnamed organisation in 2024, but that did not happen.[37]

For the time being, if you have suffered a scam and live in England, Wales or Northern Ireland, the police and agencies such as the National Crime Agency will tell you to report to Action Fraud (0300 123 2040). Scotland, however, has withdrawn from Action Fraud. You should report to Police Scotland directly, calling 101.

If you report a fraud to the local police, you will be commonly referred on to Action Fraud. Or you can report direct to them. Action Fraud may also suggest that you report to other agencies, such as HMRC.

Action Fraud's website actionfraud.police.uk tells victims of crime what Action Fraud is and how to report a crime:

We provide a central point of contact for information about fraud and financially motivated internet crime. People are scammed, ripped off or conned every day and we want this to stop.

The service is run by the City of London Police working alongside the **National Fraud Intelligence Bureau** *(NFIB) who are responsible for assessment of the reports and to ensure that your fraud reports reach the right place. The City of London Police is the national policing lead for economic crime.*

Report fraud and cybercrime
You can report fraud or cybercrime using our **online reporting service** *any time of the day or night; the service enables you to both report a fraud and find help and support. We also provide help and advice over the phone through the Action Fraud contact*

centre. You can talk to our fraud and cybercrime specialists by calling **0300 123 2040**.

When you report to us you will receive a police crime reference number. Reports taken are passed to the National Fraud Intelligence Bureau. Action Fraud **does not investigate** the cases and cannot advise you on the progress of a case.

The key to all of this lies in the last words which they emphasise in bold. Despite its title, Action Fraud **does not investigate** cases. It receives reports of crime, assesses them and in some cases passes them on to the National Fraud Intelligence Bureau (NFIB) and to the police for investigation. But there is no information as to how many and for what reasons the vast majority of cases are filtered out at each stage. *Which?* has suggested, for example, that initial reports to Action Fraud are filtered out in the first place by artificial intelligence.[38]

Not all has gone well. An undercover investigation by *The Times* newspaper in 2019 claimed that the system was not working effectively, not for victims at least. Action Fraud is funded by the Home Office and overseen by the City of London Police, but the call centre and computer systems are outsourced to a private company, not information instantly accessible on Action Fraud's website.

Information passed on to the City of London Police is, according to Action Fraud, investigated in one in four cases. According to *The Times* investigation, however, that ratio was more than optimistic, with as few as one in 50 crimes reported leading to a suspect being arrested. Many reported crimes were classified by the staff at the call centre as 'information reports' and not 'crime reports'. 'Information reports', millions of them, were kept on the computer system, for possible cross-referencing later, but most were just left on file, with no action taken. Some staff did not take reports of crime seriously, referring to some victims as 'morons'. There was also a suggestion that staff were trained to mislead victims into believing their reports would be investigated, whereas most were just left on file.

Priti Patel MP, the then Home Secretary, was 'concerned' about the findings. Meg Hillier MP, Chair of the House of Commons

Public Accounts Committee, said these revelations were 'shocking ... a let-down for all victims'.

Hopefully, Action Fraud may have improved its systems since then. The City of London Police has described it as 'the envy of police forces around the world'. Nevertheless, it is still much criticised. The Justice Committee of the House of Commons described it as 'unfit for purpose'[39] and it has been 'commonly derided'.[40] The government itself has referred to its 'shortcomings.[41] Trustpilot gives it a one-star rating.[42]

In May 2023, the then Home Secretary Suella Braverman announced that Action Fraud would be replaced by a 'state-of-the-art' reporting system by May 2024. That has not happened; the proposed replacement system remains unnamed. It will also still only be a reporting system. The Home Secretary also announced the launch of a new National Fraud Squad with 'over 400 new specialist investigators'.[43] That has not happened yet either.

Report to the National Cyber Security Centre

If you still have any energy and inclination left, report scam emails, texts and websites to this government agency (which collates data): see ncsc.gov.uk.

Property Alert

If you own a property (and particularly if there is no mortgage and you do not live there yourself), you can sign up to HM Land Registry's alert service at gov.uk, Property Alert, to get warnings of any fraudulent activity relating to your title.

Fraud and deceit abound in these days more than in former times.

Edward Coke, *Twyne's Case* (1601)

The Cost of Fraud

Fraud is now the most commonly experienced crime in the UK, **'typically targeted at elderly and other vulnerable people**, for whom the consequences can often be devastating – psychologically as well as financially'.[44]

In addition to the commonly practised frauds listed above, there are other types of fraud, too many to mention in detail – from pyramid schemes (gifting or blessing circles) to slimming scams, from charity donation frauds to tabnabbing (a phishing attack on inactive tabs left open in a browser). And there will always be new ones to keep an eye out for.

There are an estimated 3.7 million incidents of fraud each year, over 40% of all crime. One in 15 adults are the victims of fraud each year, 18% of them more than once. 41% of people over 50 are said to have been victims of fraud. The loss reported by victims overall is £2.35 billion a year.[45]

In the light of these statistics, there can hardly be any good news for older persons, although some surveys do suggest that it is the 35–44 age group that is worst hit by fraud, with the over 65s slightly less likely to be the victims of fraud and the over 75s least likely to be.[46]

You are 35 times more likely to be the victim of fraud than of robbery, ten times more than theft from the person.[47] Only one in seven of fraud incidents is reported to the police or Action Fraud, and almost one quarter of victims get no reimbursement.[48] Only 2% of police funding is dedicated to combatting fraud despite it accounting for 40% of reported crime.[49] Worse still, only a tiny proportion of incidents results in a criminal charge, just over 0.1%.[50]

Fraud (including cybercrime[51]) is a big industry and one which won't go away, although there are some signs that fraud offences are decreasing or, at least, not increasing substantially overall.[52] It is particularly big online and on social media, and in computer misuse, with fraudsters often overseas and beyond the reach of our law. 70% of fraud is said to originate abroad or have an international element.[53]

In view of the sheer numbers of fraud offences, an efficient and effective police investigation resource needs to be available for victims at all times. The Sunak Conservative government launched a *Fraud Strategy* in 2023, aiming to reduce fraud by 10% by the end of 2024. It remains to be seen what the Starmer government will do.[54]

Fraudsters are cruel and indifferent to the damage they cause. For the individual victim, particularly for the elderly, it is not just the loss of money (which can sometimes be substantial), it is the loss of confidence, of self-esteem, and, quite simply, the loss of faith in human nature. This can be devastating and not easily recovered from.

So we all need to be vigilant, both for ourselves and for those we look after. We need to look out for fraud. Most of us have been targeted in one way or another.

Fraud is certainly scary. But take heart. It can be avoided by taking simple steps and being aware.

Top Ten Tips:
What to do? What not to do?

1	**Be wary of giving your bank details to anyone,** and do not give your bank PIN number or password to anyone for any reason
2	**Check your bank accounts, including cards, very regularly (even daily) to check there are no unusual payments.** If you find any, call the bank immediately.
3	**Protect your email and bank accounts with strong and separate passwords.** Install the latest security software (e.g. anti-virus) and update apps and use two-factor authentication (if available).
4	**If anyone phones you out of the blue about investments or pensions or payments or money, put the phone down – their call is likely to be a scam**
5	**If you are offered a deal or investment that sounds too good to be true, it probably is – ignore it**
6	**If you are offered a tax rebate from HMRC by phone or email, double check it.** HMRC should have your bank details: they will not need to ask for them. The same goes for any offer suggesting you are owed or have won money.
7	**If you receive a call or email or text stating that you owe money, eg to HMRC or for a TV licence, be wary – it may well be a scam.** Check your records, call the agency and double-check the authenticity.
8	**Do not open inviting-looking emails or direct mailings online from companies you have had no dealings with** and never click on suspicious links – they may be infected with a virus so that a fraudster can hack into your account.
9	**Be wary of requests to pay by cash,** particularly for big sums, and look out for pressure to act quickly
10	**Check and double check, consult a trusted a friend or relative and if you're still in doubt, don't do it**

CHAPTER 6

Health

I am declined into the vale of years.

Shakespeare, *Othello* (1604)

Everyone knows that keeping healthy is good for life at any age. Keeping as healthy as possible at an older age is even more important. It is good for the mind and the body and for overall wellbeing, that all important feel-good factor.

But, let's face it, from time to time we all worry about the possibility of illness in later years. We know that there is a risk that we may face heart disease, stroke, cancer, diabetes, dementia (including Alzheimer's disease), Parkinson's, arthritis or osteoporosis (or something else). That's why, as individuals, we need to do as much as we can to reduce that risk.

You may be very fit for your age. You may not be. You may have let things slip a bit. But, on the positive side, there is plenty that can be done. Research indicates that **'it is never too late to look after your health and improve your chances of a healthy and independent later life'**.[1] That is why I want to summarise in this chapter some of the positive steps that research shows can be taken (if you wish). Healthy exercise, a good diet, mental and social activity, modest (or no) alcohol consumption and no smoking are central to a better life, as we all know. And much more, too.

I am not a medical person. If you need medical advice seek it professionally. I am not a personal trainer or a dietician. But there is plenty of research and information from all such experts on the best way to keep active and healthy which I want to pass on. What to do. What not to do.

For a start, have **regular check-ups** and **blood tests**. Check your blood pressure, blood sugar levels, cholesterol and other potential warning signs, including for men, a PSA blood test for prostate cancer. Then see what you can do next.

Much of this will be familiar to many of us. Quite a bit is not new, but still instructive. For example, a very well-known study, the Caerphilly Cohort Study, ran for 35 years (until 2014). It produced impressive results for participants who followed at least four of the following five guidelines:

- walk two miles or cycle ten miles, five days a week
- eat a healthy diet (including a lot of fruit and vegetables)
- maintain a healthy weight
- avoid smoking
- don't drink to excess

The results showed delayed medical conditions and a reduced risk of developing them. Those who contracted heart disease, for example, developed it 12 years later than their peers, and dementia six years later (a 60% reduced risk of dementia). They cut their chances of cancer by two thirds and diabetes by a half.[2]

As a starting point for this chapter, this study sets out a sensible framework for considering health and lifestyle in a beneficial way. There will come a time when a programme for healthy living is matched to each of us individually by genetic profiling. But not yet. In the meantime, we can take a few steps in the right direction. You may be hugely active. You may not be. I am not assuming one or the other. If what I say fits, good. If not, please move on.

New York. I almost bump into an aged New York lady as I come into the grocery store and she comes out. 'Oh sorry,' she says. 'I zigged when I should have zagged'.

Alan Bennett, Diary entry (29 October 2007) for London Review of Books Diary for 2023

Physical Activity

We all know that exercise is good for us. Research says that **all forms of exercise and activity are good**. You should do whatever suits you. Anything from working out in the gym to swimming, running, cycling, walking, exercises, lifting weights.

Gyms don't, however, suit everybody. Me included. But there are many other forms of exercise which work well. The NHS, for example, has ten-minute home workouts or the more extensive twelve-week fitness plan. YouTube has many free videos, with workouts for beginners upwards.

The NHS advises adults over 65 to aim for a minimum of two and a half hours exercise a week of moderate intensity, preferably something every day.[3] Moderate intensity exercise is described as exercise which is enough to make you breathless, such as cycling or brisk walking. If you can then move on to higher intensity exercise, so much the better. Physical activity of this kind, says the NHS, can improve your health and reduce the risk of heart disease and stroke.

Official exercise targets suggest that only bursts of activity longer than ten minutes count. But others have found from research that even shorter bursts can be beneficial.[4] Public Health England encourages at least ten minutes' walking a day. The World Health Organisation suggests at least 150 minutes of moderate intensity exercise a week to cut chances of an early death.[5] Sitting down for long periods puts the heart at risk, leads towards being overweight and to having excess blood sugar.[6]

One research study suggested that exercise for even just one hour a week can reverse mental decline. A regular exercise regime can 'turn back the clock on ageing'.[7]

Core strength is said to help delay frailty. The core is the group of muscles (abdominal, back, buttock, pelvic floor) that work together to help maintain good posture and increase stability of the spine. Pilates is popular or gym work or exercises at home. And static isometric exercises, which hold the body in one fixed position, are said to be a good way to lower blood pressure: wall sits, V-sits, planks and squat holds.[8]

As an example to all of us, Dr Catherine Walter, in her seventies, is captain of Oxford University's Linacre College female powerlifting club, *The Linacre Ladies that Lift*. Their strength training includes squats, bench presses, dead lifts and overhead presses.

But this is not necessarily all about serious activity. Other physical activities are recommended, too, such as gardening or chores around the home. 'The main thing is that people get up and do something. For some people that could just be playing with your grandchildren.'[9]

To get back to my youth I would do anything in the world, except take exercise, get up early, or be respectable.

Oscar Wilde

Benefits of exercise

Exercise is a form of insurance (a partial insurance, perhaps, and certainly not a guarantee) against medical problems in older age: stroke, heart attack, even some cancers (particularly lung and bowel cancer) and the risk of diabetes. Improving fitness by as little as 3% may reduce a man's chance of developing prostate cancer by more than a third.[10] It is an activity that can provide **positive benefits**: more energy, greater endurance, fewer aches and pains, quicker recovery from illness and less inflexibility. It also helps mental agility and awareness. It counters obesity, with all its risks.

Stability and flexibility from healthy exercise help prevent falls for older persons. As we know a fall may result not just in broken bones but a loss of confidence. Being active supports balance and coordination and helps avoid falls.

Those who have long periods of inactivity, such as sitting at a desk for nine hours a day, particularly middle-aged and older people, are two and a half times more likely to die early.[11]

Good fresh-air walking is said to be a valuable aid to health. If you are in a city, walking in a park has the benefit of oxygen from the trees. You can measure your distance with phone apps, pedometers, wrist fitness bands and other aids. The British Heart Foundation lists 11 free walking apps. You can compete (or just compare) with friends, if you want to, or even with yourself, counting the steps and kilometres. You can measure three days at a time or a week at a time. See how far you can go, and feel good about it.

Some aim for the 10,000-steps-a-day target (whereas the daily average is more like 1,500). This target is said to have originated from a Manpo-Kei, a sort of pedometer used as a Japanese marketing device invented to make Japan as a nation more healthy in the run-up (or should that be walk-up?) to the Japanese Olympics in 1964.

One study suggests that every extra 1,000 steps a day cuts the risk of dying by 16%.[12] Even a 35 minute stroll every day may reduce the risk of a stroke.[13] Others say that quick walking is good, preferably bursts of quick walking, at least walking fast enough to keep talking but not singing.

One way or another, whether by modest exercise or more energetic aerobic activity, the aim is to get our hearts beating faster for a short while than when at rest, so as to reduce high blood pressure and increase the health of the heart. According to the NHS, exercise reduces the risk of coronary heart disease, stroke, type 2 diabetes and cancer; it lowers the risk of early death by up to 30%.[14] The World Health Organisation also states that physical activity can reduce symptoms of depression and anxiety, enhance brain health and improve overall wellbeing.[15]

Mental Activity

Seneca reported on his frequent visits to a friend. 'I went to see Aufidius Bassus, a very noble fellow, stricken and struggling with his advancing years. But already there is more to weigh him down than lift him up, for old age is leaning upon him with its huge weight, everywhere ... But our friend Bassus stays sharp minded. Philosophy furnishes him with this: to be cheerful when death comes into view, to stay strong and happy no matter what one's bodily condition, and not to let go even when one is let go of ... It's a great thing, and always to be studied: when that inescapable hour arrives, go out with a calm mind.'[16]

Work and other activities

Many of us over retirement age continue to work in some form or another, usually, but not always, out of choice (**see pp 65–66**). I am lucky enough to have that opportunity. Many volunteer for charities and other organisations. Many are active (physically and mentally) as carers, for the elderly, for partners and for grandchildren, which are invaluable, if exhausting, jobs.

Many of us are familiar, too, with the range of post-retirement activities that are available to us: exercise or specialist gym programmes; intellectual, musical and artistic endeavours; and, of course, everyday mind activities, such as puzzles,[17] that stimulate the brain. All offer physical or mental stimulus and the positive benefits of sociability. Social relationships benefit both mental and physical health.[18]

One author encourages the retired not to drift through retirement but to plan for it, working hard on giving life a new purpose. 'We shouldn't fear it – we should embrace it.'[19]

Do you think my mind is maturing late,
Or simply rotted early?

Ogden Nash, *Lines on Facing Forty* (1942)

Diet

We all know that healthy eating is good for us and is conducive to better living when we get older. I am not going to tell you what to eat. You are old enough to know better. But I will make some suggestions for healthy eating, based on what experts have concluded. All the research confirms that **healthy eating** provides energy for an active life, reduces excessive weight, provides variety for the gut and lessens the risk of serious illness.

By diet, I mean food. I don't mean dieting. Although if you want to lose a little extra weight then there will be a 'diet' somewhere for you. I do not propose to advise on diets or fasting. Please note that the British Dietetic Association has advised avoiding any 'diet' that aims to offer a quick-fix weight-loss solution. They may work at first, but then lead to yo-yo weight increase and muscle loss.[20]

Some experts warn against diets because we all respond to food in different ways and at different times of the day, so that one diet may work for one person but not for another.[21] The variation from one person to another is said to be partly genetic, partly dependent on the microbes in the gut. For this reason, the more diverse your diet, with the necessary inclusion of fruit and vegetables, nuts, olive oil and pulses, plus fibre and polyphenols, the more diverse your microbiome will be.[22]

There are, of course, good reasons for a healthy diet. In the UK almost two thirds of adults are estimated to be overweight, with 27% of them obese. Those aged 65 to 75 have more obesity than any other age group.[23] According to Cancer Research UK, obesity is the second biggest cause of cancer in the UK.[24]

Turning to a healthier diet will lead not just to weight reduction. It will provide added energy to stay active in later life and help reduce the risk of type 2 diabetes and heart disease.[25] Fat but fit is said to be 'a myth'. According to one study, obese women who are otherwise healthy are 39% more likely to suffer heart problems.[26]

Good for you

It's not too late, the experts say. Even modest changes in the right direction will help.

Eat regular meals, the experts say. Don't snack too much. And eating slowly helps too. Slow eaters, it has been suggested, are over 40% less likely to be overweight than fast eaters.[27]

The following foods are **generally recommended**[28]:

- fish (and chicken)
- fresh fruit
- fresh vegetables (particularly leafy greens such as spinach and kale; beetroot)
- nuts (cashews, hazelnuts, brazils, almonds, pistachios)
- mushrooms
- strawberries, blueberries (all berries, whether frozen or fresh)
- lentils, beans, chickpeas
- olive oil

Even coffee can be put on the list, according to a number of studies, even as much as two to three cups a day (three to five cups in one study), although not what you could put in it such as sugar, syrups, cream and toppings. Coffee contains antioxidants which are linked to a reduced risk of cardiovascular disease.[29] Some experts suggest that moderate amounts of coffee, dark chocolate, high fat yoghurt, wine and cheese (especially traditional cheese not synthetic varieties) may actually be 'likely to be healthy'.[30]

Drinking plenty of water is also recommended.

The so-called Mediterranean diet is much hyped. It consists mainly of the recommended foods in the list above and is said to reduce the risk of heart disease, diabetes and cancer. At the very least it can improve mood, research shows, even help depression. It can also lead to weight reduction. One study from the extensive UK Biobank concluded that the Mediterranean diet coupled with a healthy 'Mediterranean lifestyle' (an active and social life, with adequate rest such as naps) could reduce the risk of all-cause premature death. Another study found the diet was associated with healthy brain ageing.[31]

Critics of the Mediterranean diet are few and far between. They point to the possibility of weight gain from eating fats in olive oil and nuts, to low levels of iron and calcium (little dairy) and the regular consumption of wine. But this disparagement seems to be heavily outweighed by evaluations in favour.

To the list above could be added cereals and cereal products such as wholegrain bread, pasta and brown rice. A good diet of these products, with moderate portions of fish, white meat and some dairy products, but not red meat, not too many carbohydrates and not too much dairy, tends to reduce the risk of developing type 2 diabetes, high blood pressure and high cholesterol.[32] Eggs are nutritious, too, (vitamins and protein), with previous scares about cholesterol now generally thought to be unfounded.

It will be your choice, of course, whether you eat meat, poultry, fish or dairy. Vegetarian, vegan and pescetarian are all choices. We are all different.

One study found that an intake of over 25 grams of fibre a day reaped the most health rewards and could result in a decrease by 15 to 30% in 'all-cause and cardiovascular-related mortality'. It recommended increasing the daily intake of fibre, with more unprocessed wholegrains such as wheat, oats, barley, brown rice, quinoa, lentils, beans and chickpeas, in addition to fruit and vegetables.[33]

Not good for you

This may be familiar territory, but it is worth remembering that nutritionists repeatedly say that **the following should be avoided**, at least in anything more than moderate quantities:

- red meat (in more than moderation)
- processed foods
- bread with preservatives (usually sliced, and avoid emulsifiers and excessive salt)
- crisps and similar products
- junk food, fatty foods
- products with sugar, including biscuits, cakes and sweets

- fizzy sugar drinks
- sports and energy drinks
- pulp-free fruit juice

Researchers do not always come up with the same conclusions about red meat and cheese. Canadian researchers have suggested that eating red meat and cheese every day is actually good for the heart, although eating a varied diet in moderation is probably the best way to look at healthy eating.[34] But on the whole, nutritionists are inclined to suggest that red meat (beef, lamb and pork) should not be eaten too often. Chicken and dairy products (milk, butter, cheese, yoghurt) are better than red meat for reducing the risk of medical problems we may face, although, particularly with dairy (which can lead to high levels of saturated fat and salt increasing the risk of heart disease through raised blood pressure), there should be **'moderation in all things'**.[35] As one expert put it: 'Meat and dairy can contribute to a healthy, balanced diet as long as they're eaten in moderation along with plenty of fruits and vegetables, pulses, wholegrains and nuts.'[36]

Fatty foods are capable of placing two types of strain on the heart. They raise levels of cholesterol, which builds up and narrows blood vessels, and they raise blood pressure.[37] Fast foods, high sugar intake and processed foods should be avoided.[38] For chocolate lovers, dark chocolate, however, has been recognised, not necessarily as good for you, but as a mood booster, with psychoactive ingredients positively affecting mood.[39]

This is not to say that you cannot eat anything on the forbidden list. One heart surgeon (in his sixties) writes in his memoir that it is not a problem drinking pints and eating burgers; it's just a question of how many. 'I take salt by the shedload'. The effect of salt on survival has not been proved, he asserts.[40] Most experts advise, however, that older people should reduce their salt intake (no more than a teaspoonful a day), so as to avoid high blood pressure, which in turn increases the risks of heart attacks and strokes.[41]

It must, of course, be recognised that older people may to some extent have different dietary needs than younger adults. The British Dietary Association (BDA), for example, highlights, in their evidence-based resource on diet for the over-65s, *Eating, drinking and ageing well* (November 2023), that food should be chosen with 'slightly more protein, calcium, folate (folic acid) and vitamin B12'. Maintaining weight, they say, is good for your health (not if you are very overweight), as is maintaining muscle. They encourage a **nutrient-rich diet** (including fruit and vegetables, carbohydrates, fibre and dairy), plenty of fluids, and regular physical activity.

And, as the BDA says, we should all take pleasure in what we choose to eat and drink.

It was my Uncle George who discovered that alcohol was a food well in advance of medical thought.

PG Wodehouse, *The Inimitable Jeeves* (1923)

Alcohol

Despite PG Wodehouse's wit, there is little doubt that consuming more than a moderate quantity of alcohol is bad for you. On the positive side, however, **reducing levels of alcohol consumption** will correspondingly reduce the risk of a range of cancers which are associated with alcohol. Heavy drinking is also linked to liver and heart disease and it is clearly bad for the brain (strokes).

Recommended levels of consumption

The UK government recommended levels of alcohol consumption were updated in 2016. The change made then was that the recommended level for men was reduced to the same as women, namely 14 units per week. The government does not recommend drinking; it recommends a maximum level of drinking a week.

Recommended maximum levels of alcohol consumption per week

	MEN	WOMEN
Before 2016	21 units	14 units
From 2016 and current	**14** units	**14** units

14 units is approximately:

- 6 pints of average strength beer (4% strength)
- 6 medium glasses (175ml) of wine (13% strength)
- 14 measures (25ml) of spirits (40% strength)

It is also recommended that drinking should be spread across the week and not 'saved up' and drunk all at once. Avoid binge drinking. **Alcohol free days** are recommended as a good way to reduce intake.

The NHS suggests that drinking less can be a really effective way to improve your health, boost your energy, lose weight and save money.

Not all countries recommend levels of consumption in terms of units. Counting by the number of maximum drinks recommended each week is now more common. So, if the UK's 14 units a week (for men and women), which is similar to Italy's and Germany's 14 units for men (although less for women in both countries, seven units), is translated as roughly six drinks a week (men and women), the following comparisons with the current recommended maximum levels in some other countries can be made:

- Netherlands: 7 drinks (men and women)
- France, Denmark, Australia: 10 drinks (men and women)
- Finland, Greece, USA: 14 drinks (men), 7 drinks (women)
- Canada: 15 drinks (men), 10 drinks (women)
- Ireland: 17 drinks (men), 11 drinks (women)
- Belgium, Switzerland, New Zealand: 21 drinks (men), 14 drinks (women)

I'm on a whisky diet. I've lost three days already.

Tommy Cooper

Spain and Norway both measure recommended levels not by units or drinks, but by weight of alcohol (140gms for men, 70gms for women). This approximates to ten and a half drinks (men) and five drinks (women).

There is plenty of evidence that **drinking alcohol more than moderately can damage health**, with research findings that heavy drinking increases the risk of dementia, higher than smoking or high blood pressure. It has been described as 'a major risk factor for all types of dementia'.[42] The Medical Research Council has found that alcohol can cause cancers by permanently damaging stem cell DNA.[43]

And there is plenty of evidence that consumption in the UK is too high. Alcohol-related deaths are on the increase in the UK. More than 10,000 people die each year from wholly related alcohol-specific causes (higher in Northern Ireland and Scotland).[44] Cancer Research has estimated that alcohol contributes to 12,000 deaths a year in the UK.[45] One piece of research, for example, on 28,000 people aged over 65 living in London, found that one in five was consuming at an unsafe level. Men were 65% of these unsafe drinkers.[46]

But following government guidance, or drinking less, will undoubtedly be a help. Cutting down, if you are already a drinker, may help you live longer. This was the conclusion of one of the biggest studies in this field. Six hundred thousand drinkers from 19 countries, mostly in the UK, were followed up for 30 years. The risk of dying early started to increase if more than about 100g of alcohol a week was drunk. This is the equivalent of 12 and a half units (less than the recommended maximum), which the study said increased the risk of stroke by 14%.[47]

On the other hand, and I would add a note of caution, some research has concluded that moderate consumption may not do any harm, and may even do some good. One study suggested that middle-aged moderate drinkers are about one third less likely to have a heart attack than those who have always been teetotallers. Another study concluded: 'Infrequent, light, or moderate drinkers [as opposed to 'heavy drinkers'] were a lower risk of mortality from all causes.'[48] Alcohol, to that extent, may have a protective effect, particularly in women. But it should be firmly noted that other, previous, studies found that any benefit for the heart was outweighed by a higher risk of strokes, cancer and vascular dementia.[49]

The extolling of the virtues of wine in a whole chapter in the 16th-century *Secreti Eccellentissimi Huomini del Mundo*, stating that it chases away melancholy, fights off quatrain fever, purges bad blood, cures fistula and ensures a clear complexion for women, should perhaps be taken with a pinch of salt.

Some research has suggested that red wine, not other types of drinks, may have benefits. It may help the gut and reduce levels of bad cholesterol and obesity. Red wine is said to contain many polyphenols, antioxidant defence chemicals which are to be found in many fruits and vegetables and tea. They are said to provide a healthy mix of bacteria in the gut which may boost the immune system. This does, of course, refer to moderate red wine drinking, with even just one glass every two weeks producing a positive effect, or, in another study, 'every now and again'.[50] Rather limited grape expectations.

One correspondent wrote to a national newspaper, suggesting (with tongue in cheek and possibly glass in hand) what she hoped the paper would publish in her 99th year: 'Scientists finally prove that red wine is the secret to longevity.'

On the other hand, a study of studies has recently concluded that there is simply no completely 'safe' level of drinking.[51]

Age appears to be best in four things: old wood to burn, old wine to drink, old friends to trust and old authors to read.

Francis Bacon, *Apophthegms New and Old* (1625)[52]

Smoking

Don't. If you smoke, give it up. It is a deadly killer.

The World Health Organisation (WHO) states that tobacco kills up to one half of its users, some eight million people a year world-wide, including an estimated 1.3 million non-smokers who are exposed to second-hand smoke.[53] Cancer Research UK states that smoking remains the biggest single cause of cancer, with an estimated 55,000 deaths a year in the UK, killing one person in the UK every five minutes.[54]

Nevertheless, smoking numbers are reducing and smokers are smoking less. In 2023, nearly 12% of all adults in the UK smoked, around 6 million people (those in the over-65 age group had the lowest proportion of smokers, about 8%). This figure reduces year by year and is down 8% since 2011. Average daily consumption of cigarettes is down too, from 13.8 cigarettes a day (in 2000) to 10.6 a day (in 2022). England has the lowest proportion of smokers of the four nations, with men more likely to smoke than women, and those defined as unemployed more likely to smoke than those in paid employment.[55]

Contrary to popular belief, smoking may also increase levels of fat, known as 'visceral fat', which is linked to increased levels of heart disease, diabetes, stroke and dementia.[56]

Sleep

Good sleep, researchers suggest, is on a par with good diet and good exercise.[57] It also has a positive effect on your diet, by reducing the number of calories you feel you need.[58] Seven or eight hours of sleep should be the target. It recharges your batteries.

Although this may sometimes become more difficult as we get older, good sleep may reduce the risk of heart attack, stroke and other major diseases substantially. A poor night's sleep, on the other hand, may affect adversely the brain's capacity to learn and function cognitively by as much as 40%.[59]

A short – and the emphasis is on short – daytime nap, maybe 20 minutes, may help 'preserve the health of the brain' and im-

Sleeping is no mean art; you need to stay awake all day to do it.

Friedrich Nietzsche

prove cognitive performance as we get older (although there is also some limited negative research on naps).[60]

Sleeping pills should be used only in the short term. One study found links (which are not necessarily the same as causation) between taking sleeping pills and earlier death, including cancer.[61]

As you will know, if you have difficulty sleeping the usual things are to be avoided: coffee (even decaffeinated), tea and alcohol. We should **keep hydrated**; drink more water through the day.[62] Some other products may contain caffeine, such as chocolate and cocoa drinks. And some medics advise that tea and coffee should be avoided any time after lunch. They dehydrate you. Water is better. Others say avoid them after five pm or so.

More than five hours of TV a day is 50% more likely to get you up at night (nocturia).[63] Screens should be avoided late at night.[64] And work should be kept out of the bedroom.[65] Research shows that the body and the brain need to know that a change is coming, that you are getting ready to sleep. It's a question of setting the clock to distinguish between day and night, even a regular going-to-bed time and routine.

Some say that it makes it easier to sleep if you clear the mind before going to bed by writing out a to-do list for the next day or writing down your worries and concerns.[66]

The following **recipe for good sleep**, sometimes called 'sleep hygiene', has been prescribed by one expert[67]:

- Sleep on a good bed/mattress
- Go to bed and get up at roughly the same time each day
- Avoid binge sleeping
- Sleep in a room which is cool[68] (and calm); open the window
- Sleep in the dark

- Dim the lights towards bedtime (conversely, have strong daylight in the morning)
- Avoid screens before bedtime, especially close to the eyes; keep TV out of the bedroom
- Avoid work shortly before bedtime
- Exercise during the day, but not just before bedtime
- Do not nap for too long during the day
- Avoid caffeine (tea, coffee) in the hours before bedtime
- Avoid food for two to three hours before bedtime, but do not go to bed hungry
- Eat a diet high in fibre and low in sugar
- Avoid alcohol shortly before bedtime

Some experts, however, say that this kind of list is unnecessary. We are all different and will have different sleep needs. Therefore we can condition ourselves to sleep contrary to some suggestions on the list. It is up to you. What works best for you is best for you. Some favour yoga and meditation or breathing exercises. If you have a bad night's sleep, try not to worry too much. Sleeplessness happens. It should not become a great worry in itself.

Wellbeing

We must be getting something right. The Office for National Statistics (ONS) suggests that residents in the UK who are 65 or over are happier, less anxious and have a greater sense of self-worth than all other age groups. ONS added: 'Contrary to a commonly held belief that ageing involves loss and increasing burden, those aged 65 and older are currently faring better on many measures of personal, social and financial wellbeing than their younger counterparts.' Those still working at 75 report the greatest level of job satisfaction of all ages. The 75 and older age group is more likely to be satisfied with their income, leisure time, feel they can cope financially and belong to their neighbourhood than any other age group. Engaging in a socially active life is associated with higher late-life wellbeing.[69]

There are many routes to wellbeing. The Japanese have a method called *Shinrin-yoku*, literally bathing in the forest: walking in woodland, breathing deeply and contemplating nature calmly. A stroll in the park was described by one researcher as a 'nature pill', a low-cost remedy for various health issues including high blood pressure and mental illness.[70] Trees absorb pollution in the air and give off fresh oxygen in return. A green park, and most of them are green, is said to lift your mood, particularly with plenty of trees. Listening to birdsong is also good.[71]

The right sort of indoor plants can help, too. It is said that plants such as African violets and devil's ivy give off hydrogen peroxide. They can help 'disinfect air' and protect from colds and flu.[72] Read about healthy indoor plants in *Spruce up your home, p 219*.

Whether you choose some form of mindfulness, meditation, yoga, hygge,[73] retreat, reflection or just relaxation, there will be something that works for you, something that reduces stress and anxiety.

One study found that as many as 43% of people believe that stress causes cancer. There is no evidence to support this theory, although stress is known to affect the immune system. The study did, however, suggest that about four in ten cancer cases could be prevented through improved lifestyle changes.[74]

Retirement presents delights and challenges. For many it is a release after a lifetime of work. It is a time to take up hobbies and pastimes; an opportunity to help out the family (grandchildren). We know we confront a number of losses: loss of income, status, sense of purpose, the camaraderie of colleagues, a structure to our day. Overall, that can engender a lack of self-respect. Well-being tactics may need to be deployed. Some people just have to be active. Others need to be more reflective. There are plenty of local opportunities for both.

It is beautiful to see a human being pass across the motionless face of nature without disturbing it.

Simone de Beauvoir, *Force of Circumstance* (Penguin, 1976)

Dementia

It is not the purpose of this book to look at all different kinds of illnesses, ailments and conditions which afflict (I could think of stronger words) people in older age. The words 'old age' and 'infirmity' too often go together. But no book about older people would be complete without some mention of dementia.

And dementia may well affect *mental capacity*, in its legal sense, the ability to take rational decisions about money, property, health, care and resuscitation, which was discussed in Chapter 1 in the context of *Advance Decisions* (living wills) and *Lasting Powers of Attorney* (**see pp 19, 31**).

The bad news

The bad news is bad. Not only are the numbers of dementia sufferers increasing, but dementia has also risen up the list of causes of death.

There are said to be nearly 950,000 people (on some figures, one in 11 of those over 65) in the UK suffering from dementia, a figure expected to rise to a million by 2030 and 1.6 million by 2050.[75]

The leading cause of death in England and Wales, identified by the Office for National Statistics in broad disease categories, is dementia and Alzheimer's disease (11.6% of all registered deaths), closely followed by ischaemic heart disease (10%).[76] In the later stages of dementia, the decline in brain function may lead to complications and infections, such as pneumonia.

WHO, on the other hand, has dementia as the seventh leading cause of death (1.8 million people worldwide), with women disproportionately affected. Heart disease, Covid-19 and stroke are the first three on the WHO list.[77]

*Old age is, so to speak,
the sanctuary of ills: they
all take refuge in it.*

Antiphanes, *Fragment* (c.350 BC)

The good news

The good news for the over 65s is that the risk of developing dementia can be reduced, to some extent at least. Once the risk factors are clearly identified, steps can be taken to alleviate them. **The risk factors** usually associated with dementia are diabetes, high blood pressure, and raised cholesterol. One study also suggested avoiding traffic pollution. Smoking and alcohol are also on the list, as is obesity.[78]

Research on older people in the UK suggests that a high level of muscle strength may make it 26% less likely that Alzheimer's and Parkinson's will develop, with a 13% lower likelihood if substantial fat around the stomach and arms is reduced. (By contrast, one piece of extensive research, controversially and contrary to other studies, suggests that being overweight can cut the risk of dementia.[79])

These high-risk factors can, however, be managed and reduced by a healthy lifestyle. Since there is no cure, reducing the risk of dementia by improving lifestyle seems to be our only way forward.

It is certainly not all gloom and doom. Bill, 71, married his girlfriend Anne, 69. Nothing unusual about that. The difference is that Bill and Anne were already married, to each other, and had been for 12 years. Suffering from dementia, with severe memory loss, he was convinced that Anne was his new girlfriend. He asked her to marry him and she agreed. And he did not forget. He kept asking when they would be married. They had a second wedding, renewing their vows. Anne described it as a 'most beautiful day', with friends and family gathered together to celebrate. Hopefully for Bill it was magic too. He used to be a magician with his own show on Grampian TV in the 1990s.[80]

What is dementia?

Dementia is variously described as a condition or a disease or a syndrome. It is often described as a syndrome associated with an ongoing decline of brain function. Typically, it starts with a decline in short-term memory. It can also affect the way people think, speak, perceive things, feel and behave.

WHO describes dementia in these terms:

Dementia is an umbrella term for several diseases affecting memory, other cognitive abilities and behaviour that interfere significantly with a person's ability to maintain their activities of daily living. Although age is the strongest known risk factor for dementia, it is not a normal part of ageing.

Dementia takes many forms, such as mixed dementia, vascular dementia, dementia with Lewy bodies and frontotemporal dementia disease. Alzheimer's disease is the most common form, 60 to 70% of all dementia cases in the UK (mostly those over 65).[81] Alzheimer's disease is a progressive condition which affects multiple brain functions. As the condition develops, memory problems become more severe and other symptoms, such as confusion, disorientation, speech problems, difficulty with everyday tasks and personality changes, may develop.[82]

Symptoms

The NHS explains dementia in this way:[83]

Dementia is a syndrome (a group of related symptoms) associated with an ongoing decline of brain functioning. This may include problems with:

- *memory loss*
- *thinking speed*
- *mental sharpness and quickness*
- *language*
- *understanding*
- *judgement*
- *mood*
- *movement*
- *difficulties doing daily activities*

Even before a clear diagnosis of dementia, the following are some common early symptoms at a practical level:

- memory loss
- difficulty concentrating
- difficulty with ordinary daily tasks (such as getting confused over change when shopping)
- struggling to follow a conversation or find the right word
- getting confused about time or place
- mood changes

Please don't panic. Some of these early symptoms, such as memory loss, may just be a sign of getting older. We are all inclined to forget names and other details. But if you have a doubt about yourself or a close relative, you may wish to consult a GP. An early diagnosis may make some difference. One test you can try yourself is to name as many countries (it could be fruits or animals or musical instruments) as you can in 60 seconds. A decent score is said to be 20 to 25. A not-so-good score of 10 to 15 on such tests may indicate memory difficulties.

One study, involving a modest sample, claims to have identified a technique which distinguishes between those who have the early stages of Alzheimer's disease and those who have problems from just ageing. It identifies Alzheimer's by a test which asks patients to navigate a virtual reality world using headsets. Another piece of research also favours PET brain imaging (positron emission tomography) in order to identify tau-protein 'tangles' which lead to brain degeneration.[84] It is not clear whether an early loss of hearing may be a possible indicator. But some research suggests that treating early signs of hearing loss may help ward off mental decline and that wearing a hearing aid can slow the process of dementia by up to 50%.[85]

Cure

There is no cure for dementia. Prevention and management by a **healthier lifestyle** is all that is recommended. The extent of lifestyle benefit is not, however, known precisely.

A number of drugs are being trialled to slow down the early onset of Alzheimer's disease. They include some potentially successful immunotherapy drugs, including lecanemab, donanemab and remternetug.

Lecanemab (brand name Leqembi) was licensed for use in Great Britain in August 2024, although it is not available on the NHS because the benefits were considered too small to justify the cost. Lecanemab has been shown to slow cognitive decline in some patients in the early stages of Alzheimer's. The Alzheimer's Association said: 'The treatment will allow people to have more time to participate in daily life and live independently.'[86] Donanemab (brand name Kisunla) has followed the same path. It was approved by the US Food and Drug Administration (FDA) in July 2024 for the treatment of Alzheimer's disease for patients with 'mild cognitive impairment or mild dementia', but, although now licensed in the UK, it is not 'currently' available on the NHS.

One large study suggests that a recent shingles vaccine, Shingrix (now offered on the NHS to those 65 and over), may significantly delay the onset of dementia.[87]

Management

It is important to emphasise that many people with dementia lead active fulfilled lives. But management of the condition really helps.

Studies show that a **healthy lifestyle** undoubtedly helps to manage and slow down the development of dementia. The WHO list (*see p 204 below*), for keeping dementia at bay, is a familiar list for lifestyle improvements.

Some researchers have suggested that the many cocktails of medications which some older people take for other conditions may be harmful in this context, increasing the risk of dementia. Prescriptions should be reviewed with this in mind.[88]

Help and support can be very beneficial, without taking away independence. Reassurance and support are invaluable. The effects of dementia, for example in dealing with everyday tasks, can be demoralising. The sufferer may feel isolated, anxious, even scared, so **reassurance** helps.

Encouragement with hobbies and interests will help too, especially those that are familiar to the patient. Even just one hour a week with a patient can help.[89] Remember that dementia may be followed by loneliness. Social activity is therefore important. And, as always, a healthy balanced diet helps support quality of life, with regular meals and drinking fluids a must. Being as active as possible, physically and mentally, is of particular help for the brain.

When a sufferer has difficulty explaining something, **be patient** and try to be understanding. An older person with short-term memory loss may forget what you said shortly before, but they will not forget how they *feel* you dealt with them. When someone asks you for the sixth time 'What are we having for lunch?' a kind answer said patiently and sympathetically will always help. Speaking directly with the person and listening to them directly, without distractions, will help them. Speaking about a subject you know they will be interested in, such as grandchildren, will always help. Looking at photos may be welcomed. Don't disagree too much; try not to contradict and cause worry. Keep it simple. Smile. Be positive. One to one personal contact may reduce agitation and aggression.[90]

Loss of memory may be short-term loss only. Go back over time to find subjects of interest in the long-term memory. My highly intelligent (and delightful) mother-in-law could not remember who visited half an hour ago: 'You see, my memory's gone', she would say. But on one occasion I asked her if she remembered learning to ride a bicycle. She did. She told me, with pleasure, where she did it and who helped her.

Three things happen when you get to my age. First your memory starts to go ... I've forgotten the other two.

Norman Wisdom

If you are struggling with the person you care for or visit, seek advice. Talk to family and friends. Consult organisations online.[91] Your GP could help.

One well-known dementia sufferer invited doctors to be more positive with dementia patients, trying not to give the impression that 'this is the end'. She also recommended that patients who can't read novels because of short-term memory loss should read something short: short stories, articles or poems. She also suggested practical steps, such as iPads pinging as a reminder to take pills or having a bright pink bike because it is less easy to leave behind.[92]

Many of us will be familiar with a memory box. You can put in photos, objects from the past, a letter from a loved one, a favourite soap, a preserved herb. A memory box is something to turn to and discuss.

How to avoid dementia

There is no doubt that a **healthy, active lifestyle** helps to avoid dementia. The head of research at Alzheimer's Research UK has said: 'The best evidence indicates that staying physically and mentally active, not smoking, controlling blood pressure and cholesterol, drinking only within recommended guidelines and eating a balanced diet are all linked to better brain health.'[93]

A study published in *Alzheimer's & Dementia* suggested that the most active (mentally and physically) people were 55% less likely to develop frontotemporal dementia, a common form of dementia which typically begins in the 45–65 age range.[94]

WHO has provided international **guidance for keeping dementia at bay**.[95] The list, by now, in the light of other advice, looks rather familiar:

- eat more fruit, vegetables, fish and nuts
- take less sugar and fat
- walk about for about 20 minutes a day; take at least two or three hours of moderate[96] physical activity a week
- no smoking

- cut down alcohol
- keep blood pressure and diabetes under control
- slim down if overweight

Another study concluded, positively, that a similar list can reduce the risk of dementia by 70%, even if it is started after retirement.[97]

WHO also suggested that vitamin supplements were not recommended because of side-effects. Others have suggested that aspirin is not recommended either.[98]

As we all know, a healthy lifestyle includes a healthy mental lifestyle. Those who read more (or write more), for example, have been found to have a third the risk of developing dementia. The same applies to other cognitively stimulating activities, such as playing a musical instrument, particularly the piano.[99]

A social and cultural life is recommended, maintaining friends and social networks, as well as keeping up links with younger people, including visits by grandchildren. So is just getting out and doing things. One study found that being socially active and reducing loneliness reduced the risk of dementia by 30 to 50%; social interaction helped by reducing stress and improving blood flow to the brain.[100] There is also said to be a correlation between internet use (including email) and good mental health for older people.[101]

Grieving

Death is ordinary in that it happens to us all. But its effects on those left behind are extraordinary.

The loss of a loved one is the most devastating thing that can happen to us, particularly if it is the loss of a long-term partner.

How we deal with bereavement will depend on who we are. There are many sources of help and support out there. Grieving is universal and can be protracted and painful.

It is worth remembering that loss is not confined to bereavement and we may grieve the loss of a partner through divorce or separation, the loss of a job or a home if we move.

Whoever it is or whatever it is that triggers the loss, its effects can be fundamental and we may need to acknowledge that we need help. Perhaps we older persons have the younger generation to thank for learning about the importance of being more open. Gone are the days of valuing the 'stiff upper lip'.

Many of us will be familiar with the five stages of grief identified many years ago by psychologist Elisabeth Kubler-Ross. These are denial; anger; bargaining; depression and finally acceptance.

Older people have traditionally used denial as a (useful) coping mechanism and the anger that follows can be a result of locking up the other feelings that loss triggers. What we all know is that grieving is a process and that the pain of loss will ease and abate over time.

There is help out there, particularly for bereavement. For example, the charity Independent Age offers *GriefChat*, which is a free service where you can talk to a specially trained bereavement counsellor.

Top Ten Tips: for a Healthy Life (from Expert Research)

1	Stay healthy, get healthier
2	Take regular exercise – even modest walking
3	Eat a healthy diet and watch your weight
4	Drink no alcohol or drink moderately. Follow the recommended units of consumption.
5	No smoking – it kills 50% of smokers
6	Sleep well, at least seven hours if possible
7	Keep active socially
8	Keep active mentally
9	If worried (for yourself or somebody close) about dementia, consult your GP
10	Remember the good things – the over 65s are the happiest and least anxious age group, with the greatest sense of self-worth

CHAPTER 7

Home

*I look up at the bright moon
I look down at the dark earth
And I think of home*

Li Bai (701–62), *Quiet Night Thought*

For most older people who live in their own home, staying at home for as long as possible is key. Not only is the home familiar, comfortable and much loved, but it may also be full of memories.

Many people in the UK live alone, some 8.4 million. Half of them, some 4.2 million, are aged 65 or over.[1] The circumstances of an older person may sometimes be challenging, but being able to remain at home may be a big boost, a big positive in a difficult older life. Hopefully, there are relatives and friendly neighbours, too, who will pop in and help out, if and when needed.

There are different ways of staying at home. If you are fit and active, this is no problem. But if you are less so, there may come a time when you need to make changes (either on your own or in a couple) which make living at home easier and safer.

Some of the **stay-at-home options** available include:

- making your home safer with locks and home security systems
- alarm bell and tech systems for medical emergencies
- adapting your property to make daily life easier; some of the simpler adaptations, such as ramps, handrails and lever

taps, may come free from the local council after a needs assessment
- sharing your home with a helping lodger
- having carers visit or live in

If living at home is no longer viable, you may need to **consider moving**:

- downsizing to something more manageable, especially a property without stairs
- moving to one of the several types of sheltered housing, where you are still independent but have the benefit of support services on hand; it is better to move out into something more suited to your needs before it is too late to move
- moving to a care home or care and nursing home, for 24-hour care and support

Security Measures

For safety and peace of mind make sure your property is secure. All reasonable steps should be taken to reduce the risk of theft and the opportunity for breaking in. Keep yourself safe with good locks and strong doors. Keep valuables out of reach. Watch out for unusual visitors and potential intruders.

Some of the following steps may prevent crime.

Keeping safe at home

Doors and windows	Use good locks • strong deadlocks on doors (and strong doors, particularly back doors which get neglected) • sound locks on windows Good locks may reduce insurance premiums
Points of access	Keep secure, including small kitchen and toilet windows (which some burglars favour)
Keys and valuables	Keep out of sight and of reach • away from the letter box • not just inside the front door or in a hallway • no keys under the mat, behind a plant pot or storage bin Lock valuable jewellery away
Phones, tablets and laptops	Keep out of sight, away from windows (these are attractive items to burglars)
Bicycles, etc	Keep locked and out of sight
Burglar alarm systems	Be prepared for a substantial initial outlay, plus a regular monthly payment for 'servicing'
Home security systems	Mains or battery-operated home security systems are also available, using cameras and sensors to detect unusual movement
Outside lighting	To see potential intruders To let neighbours see if anything is amiss

Video doorbell	To see who is at the door before you open it, or even to see someone who comes close to your door A visible video can also act as a deterrent (Some video doorbells require regular subscription fees)
Unexpected callers	Watch out for thieves: • getting into your home on a pretext: a glass of water, to use the toilet • using a distraction (like a chat), while a second person searches for valuables (*see pp 153–155*)
Going away	Use timer lights to suggest someone is at home Ask a neighbour to keep an eye out Install a home security system with cameras and/or motion sensors

Warning Alarms

Some alarms, such as fire and smoke alarms, are well-known essentials. Less well-known are the dangers from carbon monoxide poisoning. Carbon monoxide alarms are essential too.

Carbon monoxide

This can be deadly. Gas boilers, gas fires, open fires, wood burners, coal-fired stoves and oil heaters can all emit carbon monoxide if faulty, for example if not installed properly or poorly maintained. And the dangerous thing about carbon monoxide is that it is odourless and colourless. Leaked carbon monoxide, particularly in a confined space, can spread without you knowing. If it gets into the blood, it replaces oxygen in red blood cells, causing symptoms of headache, dizziness, nausea or vomiting, confusion, muscle pain or shortness of breath.[2] In severe cases death may result. Carbon monoxide alarms are therefore essential.

Warning alarms

Fire and smoke alarms	Essential: • make sure they are in place and working • check to see that the batteries are charged • check with your local fire service if you need advice; they will often install alarms free of charge[3]
Carbon monoxide alarms	Essential: • install an alarm in every room with a fuel-burning device (for example a gas boiler in a kitchen or bathroom) • check that each alarm is working • make sure that a gas boiler is serviced regularly by a qualified engineer • make sure all fuel-burning devices are properly maintained • keep chimneys and flues clean and well maintained • seek medical advice urgently if you suspect you have been affected by carbon monoxide poisoning; seek urgent advice to remedy the leak
	There is: • a 24-hour national gas emergency number 0800 111 999 (or text 0800 371 787) • solid fuel advice numbers 01773 835400 (also 0845 6014 406) • an OFTEC oil-fired advice line 0845 65 85 080 (also 01473 626 298) • a health and safety carbon monoxide advice line 0800 300 363 (or use the gas emergency number above) As always there are the health and emergency lines 111 and 999

Alarm Bell Systems

If you are at home but getting less mobile or otherwise feeling more vulnerable, there are steps you can take to increase your wellbeing and keep you safe. If you are on your own (a single person or a couple) you can, for example, obtain an alarm bell system which is easy to use. Other technology systems, such as 'telecare', can be used to monitor you, too, for example if you have a fall. And AI systems can also provide invaluable support in different ways.

These are some of the options:

Alarm bell systems (for emergencies)

Call bell systems (personal alarms)	Get help at home at the press of a button If you have an urgent need, eg if you fall down or become ill, you just press a red bell button (which you keep round your neck or wrist) and a call centre will speak to you through a speaker The call centre will: • ask if you need an emergency service, or • call family or neighbours (nominated by you as contacts) to check on you
Fall alarms	A similar product which also monitors with a sensor any fall and calls for help[4]
Telecare	A technology system which uses **sensors** to monitor unusual movements or when anything goes wrong (eg a fall, a spillage or the front door left open), and links to a call centre
Other alarm systems	Pull-cord alarms Gas shut-off devices

Medical Aid Systems, AI

Telehealth

This is a form of telecare (*see above*) which acts as remote medical care: you can be monitored at a distance for blood pressure, heart rate, weight and glucose levels. The local council may help with some telecare services, subject to a needs assessment.

Pill dispensers

These release medication at the appropriate time.

Voice assistants

Sometimes called voice service or virtual/intelligent/digital assistants, these include Amazon's *Alexa*, Apple's *Siri*, Google's *Assistant* and Meta's *Voicebox,* and can provide support (internet connection required). *Alexa* is the NHS's assistant of choice for delivering answers to health-related questions to smart speakers, smart phones or tablets.

These virtual assistants can:

- provide information
- make calls on request to helplines or friends and family (especially when the need suddenly arises); calling out a name to be phoned may be easier than phones with buttons
- act as medication reminders and advise when pills need to be taken (and can in some cases connect to a pill dispenser)

Remaining at Home by Adapting It

Staying at home as long as possible is usually a top priority for older people. That means that certain adjustments may need to be made. Maintaining independence, safety and comfort at home is essential.

I will turn to support from carers visiting or living-in at home in the next chapter on care (*see pp 228-238*) and I will look at options for moving out and into some form of sheltered accommodation below. But first let us consider some physical steps that can be taken to support living at home.

If you have reduced mobility, you can take steps to adapt your home to suit your needs. Walking aids and handrails, for example, can help, both inside your home and outside. These can be funded by the local authority (following a needs assessment) or privately or from charitable grants.

A needs assessment (and means test)

If you need help to cope on a day-to-day basis, the first step is to apply to your local council for *a needs assessment*. This may lead to a means test.[5] For further details, **see p 230.**

Funding

If, following a needs assessment, the council recommends equipment (such as a walking frame or personal alarm) or relatively minor adaptations (such as grab rails or a concrete ramp or steps, or lights that come on when someone is at your door), costing less than £1,000 for each adaptation, not in total, the council must provide this free of charge.[6]

In a bigger home, you can adapt your house with a stairlift or even a lift. These are expensive options, but often work well for older people. If you are in financial need, grants may be available for expensive adaptations such as stairlifts, fitting a bathroom downstairs or widening doors. Subject to income and savings, government Disabled Facilities Grants can be substantial, up to £30,000 in England, £36,000 in Wales, £25,000 in Northern Ireland. Less help is available in Scotland.[7]

The charity Independence at Home also provides grants to people of all ages with a physical or learning disability or long-term illness who are in financial need.[8] A number of charities provide free advice and more details on adaptations and products.[9]

Disabled Facilities Grants (*above*) may also help, in cases of financial need, with finance for adaptation of access to the garden and in the garden, including fitting rails and ramps and removing steps.

Adapting your home

A needs assessment	Apply to your local council, to find out what help you may need (some adaptations are free)
Alterations to property	Make life easier at home with alterations[10] such as: • handrails (grab rails), particularly in the bathroom and toilet, and on stairs • easy-to-use lever taps • adjustments in the kitchen • adjusted toilet seats • concrete ramp (instead of steps) • outside lights which come on when someone approaches
Alterations to property (in larger homes)	A stairlift (or even a lift)
Alterations to garden	If you are fortunate enough to have a garden (or a patch), you could consider making it more accessible with: • ramps (replacing steps) • wide paths • raised beds • and using specially adapted tools and equipment
	Charities such as Living Made Easy and Thrive provide good advice on help with gardening accessibility, including recommendations on tools and equipment[11]

Decluttering

This is never an easy task, particularly if your possessions harbour memories. There are home decluttering services if you want to pay for them. I try and use the three CHs: Chuck, charity or cherish. You don't have to go as far as döstädning, 'Swedish death cleaning'[12], but throwing things away that you don't need like old clothes you don't wear and piles of magazines you will never look at again could make all the difference. Don't burden your relatives with too much left behind.

There are all sorts of organisations that will help dispose of your cast-offs, particularly books and clothing,[13] in a way that produces some benefit. Your options include:

- donating to charities: shops, websites, drop-off banks
- using trade-in sites (for cash or for charity): such as sell.worldofbooks.com (books, CDs, DVDs), webuybooks.co.uk, musicmagpie.co.uk, zapper.co.uk, stuffusell.co.uk, sellitback.com, and many more
- donating to a book-sharing scheme, such as Books for London which displays books in some of London's tube and train stations
- passing on books (with special labels) and tracking their movement and readers, for example through the smart social networking site Bookcrossing.com, a US based but worldwide membership organisation
- recycling by local councils;[14] larger items may be collected (usually for a fee)
- donating to a friend or community organisation or school
- advertising locally for donation

earth after rain
old books
never read

Robert MacLean, *Wintermoon* (2022)

If you are unable to take items to a charity shop nearby, some charities and trade-in sites have free courier or drop-off services. Others offer postage alternatives.

You could declutter your garage. If you are no longer driving, give your old car to charity. Some charities accept cars which they auction or sell for scrap. Or you can donate your car to giveacar.co.uk, a not-for-profit organisation, which will sell it for the charity of your choice.

If you don't declutter, you may leave behind a troublesome burden. Will there be piles of useless stuff which relatives will have to hire a skip for? Is that fair? After all, the Swedish döstädning tells you to keep only items that are a reflection of your 'best self'. As William Morris is reported to have said, 'Have nothing in your house that you do not know to be useful or believe to be beautiful.'

Spruce up your home

Leaving aside decluttering and the cheering aspects of a lick of paint, there are important safety issues to consider at home. Make sure your carpets and floors are safe: free from obstructions, holes and not rucked up or slippery. Falls can have serious medical consequences which, sadly, can change lives.

A popular hit in Japan is Shoukei Matsumoto's book on how cleaning your house can make you happy.[15] This may not be everyone's cup of green tea, but Mr Matsumoto, who happens to be a Buddhist monk, says, 'If you live carelessly, your mind will become soiled.'

Healthy indoor plants may also help your wellbeing, particularly if mobility issues mean you get out less. House plants not only brighten up your home, they also improve the air quality. Some plants, such as spider plants, snake plants and rubber plants, absorb carbon dioxide and chemicals while replenishing the air with good oxygen.[16] Caring for your plants, keeping them alive and healthy, is also said to be positive: good for wellbeing, reducing stress and anxiety.

Accommodation Options

While we all want to live in our own home as long as possible, there may come a time when changes have to be made. Things can't go on in quite the same way as before.

Adaptations may need to be made to the property (*see above*) and other options need to be considered. These include sharing your property, care or support at home, downsizing to a smaller or more suitable property, or moving to sheltered housing. In the end, there may be no option for some but to move to a residential care home or care and nursing home.

Accommodation options

Share your home	Take in a **lodger** who, **for a reduced rent**, will help out with some of the following: • shopping for groceries • odd jobs • a little cleaning • using the computer • providing companionship The lodger, often a younger person (such as a student), can be a friend or a relative or a person matched by an agency **Matching** can be done by: • some local authorities[17] • a private or charity agency[18] The help may be ten hours a week or less. Everything should be set out in in a simple written 'licence' agreement Coupled with the government's Rent-a-Room incentive of tax-free rental income of up to £7,500 a year, this can be a helpful means of financial support[19]

Move in with a relative or friend	If they are willing, of course. But tread carefully. It may be right for you, but: • Is it right for them? • Will it work? • Are you all going to be good at sharing? • This is something that requires careful thinking and sensitive discussion It would also be sensible to have **a written agreement** to set out clearly the terms of your moving in.[20] These could include answers to these questions: • What care or support will they be able to provide? • Can the property be adapted to suit your needs? • Will you pay rent or a contribution to household bills? • If it all goes wrong, what notice should either side give for you to leave, one month, three months or six months?
Carers: visiting or living-in	These are covered in Chapter 8, *pp 228–233*
Downsize	To a smaller home or one more suitable such as one without stairs (and close to relatives and friends) **Advantages** of downsizing: • moving to a home which is smaller and therefore easier to manage • providing extra money from the sale (if you own the property, but bear in mind stamp duty) • the opportunity to declutter • freeing up a larger property for others

Older People's Shared Ownership (OPSO)	A government-supported scheme (England only) for those aged 55 or over (with gross income less than £80,000, or £90,000 in London) designed for those who can't afford to buy a home for themselves outright: you buy a part-share in a property and pay rent on the remaining share[21]
Sheltered housing (sheltered accommodation)	*see below*
Care home	This is covered in Chapter 8, *pp 236–238*

Sheltered Housing

If adapting your home or sharing or downsizing is not the right option for you, you may be ready to move to some form of sheltered housing (sometimes called sheltered accommodation).[22]

This term covers quite a wide range of housing. But usually it refers to a **self-contained individual property**, bought or rented, which is one of several linked together on one site. The property, which will often be designed especially for older people, will provide independence and privacy in your own property or unit, but it will also provide extra benefits by way of support and possibly social activities.

Sheltered housing options:

Sheltered housing	Move to a self-contained property, one of several linked together on one site. The property can be bought or rented. It is for single people or couples. The **main features** are usually: • a self-contained flat • shared communal spaces, inside and out, with shared facilities (and sometimes organised social activities) • emergency help, if required, normally available day and night • extra safety and security • maintenance and repairs on tap • a manager (or warden or officer) who can provide help The **advantages** of sheltered housing include: • maintaining a good level of independence and privacy in your own home • providing reassurance and support when needed, including emergency help • the opportunity to socialise with others if you want to
Extra care housing	This is sheltered housing plus. It is sometimes called very sheltered housing or assisted living. It offers more than the usual support and includes extra on-site services such as meals, personal care and domestic support.
Retirement home/ retirement villages	This is a variation on the same theme: • independent units on the same site • shared facilities • some sites include a care home (to move into if needed)

Close care housing	This is one step towards moving into a care home. It involves living independently in a flat on the same site as a care home. It is sometimes made available for couples with different needs.
Private or council	Sheltered housing is either private or arranged through the local council. Most councils run sheltered housing through housing associations. It is much in demand. You have to be assessed for suitability first and there may be a long waiting list. Some charities run low-cost sheltered housing.[23]
	The cost of sheltered housing varies, depending on whether you rent or buy, the scheme itself, and where you live.
	If the housing is run by the council, what you pay may depend on your means.

Outgoings	Whether you rent or buy, you will have to pay (or contribute to):
	• rent or mortgage
	• the normal outgoings such as council tax, energy bills and water charges, and (usually)
	• a service charge on the property, which covers items such as
	   – building insurance
	   – a contribution towards communal upkeep, repairs and general maintenance
	   – (possibly) payment for the manager (warden or officer) and any emergency alarm system

Prepare for a Care Home or Nursing Home

Has the time come when you can no longer manage well enough at home or in sheltered housing?

We have already looked at the various options for independent living, including living at home with support or at a different kind of property with support.[24] But there may come a time when you need to be looked after in a home. That is a difficult time. Leaving your own cherished home may be sad.

So now, the step has to be taken, by you or by somebody on your behalf, to look for a suitable care home or nursing home where you will be looked after and have 24-hour support.

More information about care and care homes is in the next chapter.

Top Ten Tips

	1	**Value the comfort and security of your own home.** Consider the options for staying at home as long as you can.
	2	**Anticipate changes in circumstances** and make changes such as adapting your home before it becomes too difficult
	3	**Keep your home safe and secure** with good locks, fire and smoke alarms and carbon monoxide alarms
	4	**Consider personal alarm systems** to deal with medical emergencies or falls
	5	**Adapt your home to your needs.** Make physical modifications, for example to deal with mobility issues.
	6	**Declutter your home and spruce it up** to make it more welcoming
	7	**Consider sharing your home.** For a reduced rent, a lodger can help out with small tasks.
	8	**Consider downsizing.** Less space will be more manageable, particularly if there are no stairs. And it might free up cash.
	9	**Consider sheltered accommodation.** Another option to ease those later years: independence plus support.
	10	**Be prepared to move to a care home or nursing home** when you need 24-hour care and support

CHAPTER 8

Care

*If I'd known I was gonna live this long,
I'd have taken better care of myself.*

Eubie Blake (1883–1983), ragtime pianist, on reaching 100

The focus of this chapter is the care of older persons. Those over 65 who need care and support in their own homes and those who reach the stage when they have to move to a care home.

Care is provided either by the state or privately. Local authorities (councils) fund and deliver state care, although most people who receive care have to make some sort of contribution to the cost. For state funding for social care, **see below**. Many older persons receiving care pay for it themselves entirely. This is known as 'self-funding'.

The complexity of care arrangements is plain to see for all those who have had direct contact with care services. As the Nuffield Trust put it: 'Navigating the social care system is highly complex and confusing.'[1]

In England alone, as many as 418,000 adults may be on care waiting lists.[2] Estimates range from 2.2 million to 4 million people aged 65 or over who have social care needs of one sort or another. And it is said that the number may rise by more than 50% within the next 20 years.[3] Figures also suggest that less than half of those with needs receive any kind of support. Of all those requesting long-term state support (including older people), the number receiving care has decreased by around 10% since 2015, and over a quarter are turned down altogether.[4]

Nevertheless, care provision is undoubtedly an extensive business. Statistics (often estimates) in this field seem to vary, but it is said that nearly a million adults in the UK receive care at home,[5] and over 400,000 are care home residents (with more than twice as many women as men).[6]

Many older persons also get help from other services such as day care, meals on wheels, home adaptations and mobility equipment.

One factor is particularly striking. Millions of older persons with needs get help, not from the state or from private services, but from **unpaid carers**, 'volunteers' of all ages, usually family or friends. And an increasing number of older persons are caring for others, too.[7] The last census in 2021 suggested there were 4.7 million unpaid carers for adults of all ages (but mostly older persons). Since then there have been estimates of 7.3 million in England,[8] even 10.6 million in the UK (59% of them women).[9]

It is not my purpose to give advice about this difficult, complex (and often controversial) topic, nor to delve into too many details. I shall just set out the key aspects of the provision of care, insofar as it affects older persons. I will look at the present system, how it works (or is intended to work), what care is available, and some of the options for change.

Home Care: Visiting Carers

Before you consider home care, you may wish to adapt your accommodation to make life easier for you at home, so that you can manage better and stay independent (*see pp 217–219*).

The next stage of support at home is visiting carers or care workers. Home care, sometimes called domiciliary care, is the provision of visiting paid carers who help you out at home, mostly with personal care.

You will probably wish to remain in your own home for as long as possible, leading an independent life. But if you need some help to manage your day-to-day living, particularly if your mobility has become restricted, home care will help you with personal care.

Home care services may include assistance with any of the following aspects of personal care[10]:

- getting up in the morning, going to bed in the evening
- washing and dressing
- using the toilet
- preparing food and drinks
- collecting prescriptions
- your medication
- shopping
- going out

You may need home care for the occasional visit or for several hours a day, depending on your needs. You may need short-term home care, for example if you have just come out of hospital, or for longer-term needs.

Who pays for home care?

Home care is hardly ever free for the person receiving it. It may be funded (usually only in part) by the state, depending on the amount of your savings. If you wish the state to pay for all or some of your care, you should apply to your local council for a needs assessment.

Whether you are likely to be state-funded or partly state-funded or not state-funded at all, you are entitled to a free assessment of your care needs from the local council. If you apply for state funding, you will need one anyway. But even if you are expecting to pay for your care yourself, a needs assessment will help provide free advice on what is best for you. For state funding for social care, *see below*.

If you receive no state funding, you will have to organise and pay for homecare yourself.

A care needs assessment

If you need help at home, you should apply to the local council for a free **needs assessment**.[11] In some areas you may have to wait a while for an assessment.[12]

The purpose of the needs assessment is to find out what, if any, help and support you need. This can include equipment for your use such as walking aids or a personal alarm, or whether you need a visiting carer for help with personal care. It can also be a **home assessment**, which will look at adaptations such as handrails and other necessary changes to your property to keep you safe and protected.

For the needs assessment you will be interviewed (face-to-face or on the phone or online) by a social worker or professional. You can have someone with you at a needs assessment to support you. The assessor may also, with your permission, contact your GP and other professionals involved in your care.

You will be asked questions about your health, how you are coping, how you manage certain physical tasks, particularly washing, dressing and cooking. This will assess the extent of the difficulties you have begun to face around the home or in your everyday actions. You should say what difficulties you have, even though they may seem trivial like having difficulty opening a cupboard. You should say what support you would like, what sort of services you need to help you.

If you are eligible for support, the council will discuss with you what services they will provide (and what services they will not), and when and how often they will be provided. There will be a care plan.

If the council decides that you are eligible for adult social care support, you will then be **financially assessed**. This is a means test (based on your income, savings and property) to see how much you can afford to contribute to the cost. This assessment is quite a complicated process and may vary from one local authority to another. It may also vary depending upon the type of service required.

Home care agencies

If you are not funded for care through the local council, you will have to organise and pay for home care yourself.

Home care agencies provide a range of services, from short visits to live-in care. There are many home care agencies to choose from.[13] You can search the NHS website for agencies in your area (in England) or there are national home care agencies.[14]

CQC ratings

All agencies in **England** must be registered with the Care Quality Commission (CQC). The CQC website, cqc.org.uk, provides information and details on each agency, including the CQC's latest inspection report and overall rating. The CQC will make an inspection for an agency (as with all adult social care services), asking five key questions. Is it:

- safe
- effective
- caring
- responsive
- well-led?

After an inspection, the CQC will provide one of four ratings, which must be displayed by the provider:[15]

- Outstanding (88–100%)
- Good (63–87%)
- Requires improvement (39–62%)
- Inadequate (38% or lower)

Check with any agency you contact that it is regulated, then double-check on the CQC website. Also check the homecare agency's rating on the helpful homecare.co.uk website.[16]

The equivalent of the CQC in **Wales** is the Care Inspectorate Wales; in **Scotland** the Care Inspectorate; and in **Northern Ireland** the Regulation and Quality Improvement Authority.

Independent care workers

Care workers (or, in some cases, nurses) working as individuals (and not employed by an agency) do not usually have to register with the CQC if the care worker works directly for you and is under your control (and is funded by you). Nor do employment agencies who supply care workers have to register, so long as they have no role in managing or directing the personal care (or nursing).[17] Unpaid carers are not required to register.

If you employ a carer directly, remember that you become an employer, with all the legal duties and responsibilities of an employer dealing with an employee. *Employing staff for the first time* on gov.uk, makes the role of an employer seem rather daunting. It suggests seven things to be done when employing someone, including checks, payment, insurance, putting the job specification in writing (with terms and conditions), and informing HMRC.[18] These seven do not include the important taking up of references.

Cost of homecare

Homecare can be provided by the local authority, if you qualify for it. First, your needs must be assessed by the council and then a financial assessment will be made by the council to assess whether you have to make a contribution to the cost. This applies in England, Wales, Scotland and Northern Ireland. For state funding for social care, *see below*.

In **England**, if you have assets of £23,250 or over, you will have to pay yourself (self-fund). Below that threshold, depending on your circumstances, you may have to make a contribution from assets or income or both.

In **Wales**, most home services involve a charge, up to a maximum of £100 a week. If you have a high income or assets in excess of £24,000 you will mostly have to self-fund. If you have less than £24,000, your income will be considered for the extent of your contribution.[19]

In **Northern Ireland**, the precise cost of home care, assessed following a care needs assessment and a financial assessment, depends on where you live and which Health and Social Care Trust you come under. Some do not charge for personal care at home.[20]

In **Scotland**, most home care is free, if you are assessed as needing certain personal care or nursing services. You may, however, have to make a contribution (following a financial assessment) for some home services, such as shopping.[21]

Care in the private sector is, of course, expensive, whether visiting care workers, live-in care workers or care in a nursing or care home. This cost may inevitably deplete savings quite quickly, particularly when living in your own home also involves the cost of running and maintaining the home, with everyday costs and expenses.

For those who are self-funding, the cost will vary. In broad terms, fees for visiting carers will be in the region of £20 to £40 an hour, on the lower side for an overnight rate (and fees may be more expensive at weekends). Live-in carer fees range from about £1,200 to £2,500 pw.

If you are not receiving benefits, you may be able to receive an Attendance Allowance or a Personal Independence Payment (formerly Disability Living Allowance) (*see pp 112-113*).

Home help

Councils, except in exceptional circumstances, do not usually fund home-help services. This kind of service, which is not usually classified as personal care, has therefore to be funded privately. Obvious services will include:

- cleaning
- washing-up
- laundry
- gardening

Different people may do different jobs. You must assess for yourself (or through a needs assessment (*above*)) exactly what help you need (what you can no longer manage sensibly on your own) and then decide who can help you. Ask around with relatives and friends for recommended people. Do not take on someone you know nothing about (*see pp 154-155*).

Unpaid carers

Unpaid carers play a significant role in caring for older persons who cannot manage so well. The term 'volunteer' may be used, but some who care for an elderly relative do not like the term 'volunteer'. They feel they have no option but to care. It may evolve organically as someone they love gradually loses the ability to care for themselves. The estimated number of unpaid carers is substantial. Details are set out in the introduction.

Carer's Allowance

There is limited funding from the state for unpaid carers. Carer's Allowance (which is gradually being replaced by Carer Support Payment in Scotland) may be available for care of an older person, as long as that person is in receipt of certain benefits. These include Attendance Allowance.

Carer's Allowance[22] is a taxable benefit of up to £81.90 per week (2024–25), rising to £83.29 (2025–2026), paid to carers (over 16 years of age) in England, Wales, Northern Ireland and Scotland. In order to be eligible to claim for Carer's Allowance:

- you, the carer, must carry out care work for at least 35 hours a week
- you must not be in full-time education, nor studying at least 21 hours a week
- if you have weekly earnings, they must be £151 or less, rising to £196 or less in 2025 (after tax, National Insurance and expenses); if you earn more one week than another, says gov.uk, *Carer's Allowance, Eligibility*, you may be able to average out your earnings, but there are some doubts about this in practice
- if you receive State Pension or benefits (such as Pension Credit (**see Chapter 3**)) or both, you cannot claim unless the amount you receive is less than £81.90 a week (Carer's Allowance may top you up to that sum)

As a carer, you can claim Carer's Allowance even if you are not related to or do not live with the person cared for. But if there is more than one carer for a cared-for person, only one carer can claim. And if you care for more than one person, you can only claim for one.

Carer's Allowance is a complex (and not exactly generous) benefit. It may even produce adverse consequences for both carer and cared-for person. Some disability-related payments and council tax reduction for the cared-for person may be put in jeopardy. And there is a risk that if the carer's benefits increase overall, the carer may move out of the threshold criteria for eligibility for Carer's Allowance and have to declare overclaiming to the DWP (not the other way round), and as a result face a heavy repayment bill.[23]

Exceptionally, the local authority may give some other kinds of support, not financial, such as help with housework or gardening or advice on benefits. You can ask for a free carer's assessment for these purposes.[24]

Respite care

Caring for an elderly person can be time-consuming, stressful, even exhausting. Unpaid carers, who are themselves often older persons (many of them women), may need a break from providing care. 'Respite care' is the term used for giving an unpaid carer a break, while the person cared for is looked after by someone else. This could be a volunteer helper, for example, or there could be a temporary place in a day centre or a care home.

Some local councils may, if you are fortunate, consider providing funding for respite care for your unpaid carer who needs a break (maybe a holiday) and provide the cared for person with temporary alternative care. The council will need to carry out both a *carer's assessment* (for the carer) and a *care needs assessment*, if not already carried out (for the cared for person), before they consider making funding available for alternative care arrangements. And all of this is means-tested too, so even if council funding is provided, a contribution may have to be made.

Some care agencies provide respite care (for a fee) for family carers. And some charities will provide free short breaks or respite funding for carers.[25]

Coming home after hospital

The hospital and local council should work together to make sure you are not discharged from hospital without the support you need at home (in theory at least). The hospital should arrange a discharge assessment or ask the council to carry out a care needs assessment (*see p 230*). You may have to pay for or contribute to the support then provided. For state funding for social care, *see below*.

Sometimes this help is not always immediately available and leads to patients staying longer than necessary in hospital when all agree they are ready to go home.[26]

Care in a Care Home

If you can no longer manage at home, even with regular care and support, one option will be to move to a care home (or nursing home). Other housing options with support are listed in Chapter 7 (*see pp 220–224*).

Care homes (and nursing homes) are either run by local councils or are private (for the self-funding). They are regulated by the Care Quality Commission (CQC). The CQC inspects and reports on care homes every year or two and provides an overall rating of each care home (outstanding, good, requires improvement, or inadequate) (*see p 231*).

Ratings and reports are published on the CQC website. They can also be found on the carehome.co.uk website.[27] **Carehome** lists residential care providers, with its own rating based on customer reviews. You can look up each care home and find extensive details under the following headings:

- Customer rating
- CQC performance rating
- Description of the property (and location) with photos
- Number of rooms, vacancies
- Type of service
- Registered and specialist care categories, such as old age, dementia
- Facilities

If you are eligible for local authority support, you have the right to choose where you live, although in practice the choices offered to you by the local authority may be limited. You may wish to visit the choices offered first.

The cost of a room in a care home or nursing home varies widely. If you are self-funding, a room in a care home will cost anything from £700 to £2,500 a week.[28] Nursing care or care in a nursing home will put up the cost. Luxury care homes cost as much as £2,000 to £3,250 a week.

Once you have decided on the move, whatever it is, relatives and friends will obviously need to help out, to make sure the change is as comfortable as possible and that you are regularly visited and called by phone. It may be a difficult time. Regular contact will be essential. For some, particularly those with dementia, who may not at the time realise exactly what is happening, continuing support from close relatives will be vital. It is also important for them to check on a continual basis that the care is appropriate, well-organised, effective and kind.

Care workers

Estimates of the number of care workers in the UK vary. The King's Fund suggests that care workers make up 860,000 of the 1.64 million filled posts in the social care sector.[29]

Care workers are not well paid, even though they may be skilled and experienced. The CQC have reported that health and care workers regularly 'fed back to us of being overworked, exhausted and stressed'.[30] (Apart from in Northern Ireland) care workers are not part of the NHS. They are paid by local authorities or care agencies or employed directly.

The work of care workers is invaluable. They work closely with the older people they look after, often carrying out intimate and sensitive work such as washing and toilet help. Their charges may have dementia. Some may be difficult. For older persons living at home, carers are sometimes the only point of personal contact on a daily basis. The work requires special personal skills. Carers need to be practical, efficient, sensitive, understanding, respectful and resourceful.

The quality of care

Much of the care provided to older persons may be excellent, although that is not always the case. According to the CQC, nearly 20% of CQC-registered 'care locations' in England require improvement.[31]

And the continuing and growing demands on care services will not help. The Department of Health and Social Care has projected that 57% more adults in England will require care in less than 20 years' time, at a cost increase of over 100%.[32]

Also, the charity Age UK has described social care for the elderly in the UK as a 'system under siege'. With an ageing population, more people with complex care needs, years of austerity, the squeeze on the budgets of local authorities, higher care costs and shortages of staff, it is a system, says the charity, with 'too much demand and too little supply'.[33]

State Funding for Social Care

The term 'social care' is usually used to include the provision of care by the state to children and adults who are vulnerable and require special care. For adults (including older persons), this includes the cost of home care or a residential place in a care home or nursing home. Local authorities (in England) spend over £24 billion a year on adult social care. Surprisingly, perhaps, only about half of that amount supports the 65 and over age group.[34] But still – a substantial sum.

In the four countries of the UK, health and social care are devolved powers (and funding). They are provided on a separate country-by-country basis. In England and Wales health care is the responsibility of central government, whereas local authorities are accountable for social care. In Northern Ireland and Scotland, health and social care are more integrated at a national level.[35]

Funding across the four countries therefore varies.

In **England**, if you have assets of less than £14,250, you may be entitled to care, whether home care or residential care, without any contribution from your assets, but you may have to make a contribution from your income. Your partner's income will not be taken into account.

If you have assets of £23,250 or more (in England), you will have to pay for your own care completely. If you have assets somewhere in between, that is between £14,250 and £23,250, you can apply to your local authority for care, but will be required to make a contribution from both assets and income.

Assets for these purposes (sometimes referred to as 'savings') include property, savings and investments. Although, if you own a property, it will not usually be taken into account if:

- you are applying for home care (ie still living at home)
- you are applying for a place in a care home, and a partner or elderly or disabled relative lives in your property
- you are applying for a place in a care home, the first 12 weeks of residence in the care home

If you deliberately dispose of any of your assets in order to reduce them so as to get care ('deprivation of assets'), they may still be taken into account by the council.

Summary: funding for care – home care and care home (England)[36]

Funding in full by the State – if assets* less than £14,250 (but with contribution from income)

Funding in part by the State – if assets between £14,250–£23,250

(with contribution from income and assets)

Private funding only – if assets more than £23,250 OR weekly income greater than care fees

* Assets = property, savings, investments

The upper limit of £23,250 has been widely criticised for being too low. It has been in place since the Care Act 2014 and has not been increased since then. The Nuffield Trust, for example, has concluded that in England: 'With consistent underfunding, access to publicly funded care for older adults is now limited to those with the lowest means and highest needs.'[37]

A higher figure of £100,000 has been proposed by various governments since 2014, but its introduction has been repeatedly postponed. It is not due to come into force, if at all, 'until October 2025' (**see below**).

Much care provision is paid, therefore, by older persons out of their own savings. Sometimes a property has to be sold to pay for long-term care. It has been estimated that four in ten adults in care homes pay entirely for themselves, a figure which rises to nearly five in ten for older people.[38] And more than a quarter of older people receiving care at home pay for it, too.[39]

Self-funders also pay more. They pay an estimated 41% more than local authorities pay for places in the same care homes.[40] An estimated total figure in excess of £8 billion is spent each year in England on privately purchased care.[41] It has been estimated that in 2010 one in ten adults aged 65 or over faced lifetime care costs more than £100,000.[42] That figure is now said to be one in seven.[43]

In **England**, care services (home care and residential care) are, therefore, rarely free. The social services departments of local authorities (local councils) provide and pay for most social care. Councils are funded largely by government grants, council taxes and business rates. They assess care needs and carry out means testing. It is estimated that nearly two million people aged 65 and over make requests of support to local authorities each year.[44]

Pressures on funding adult social care are several: a greater number of older people, increased demand for care, more complex demands for care, increases in the National Living Wage and pressure on local government finances.[45] Local authority spending on social care budgets is said to be down as much as 9% per person on the figure a decade ago, even higher in very deprived areas.[46]

Local authorities, who provide most state care, have, of course, struggled financially in recent years, with some becoming 'bankrupt'. Even before the pandemic, the National Audit Office (NAO) found in 2019 that government funding for local authorities had fallen on aggregate by 55% over a ten-year period.[47]

As a consequence, the NAO has described the adult social care sector in cheerless terms: 'The sector remains challenged by chronic workforce shortages, long waiting lists for care and fragile provider and local authority finances.'[48]

In **Northern Ireland**, the thresholds for care home funding are the same as for England, ie a maximum of £23,250. If you fall under the threshold, the local authority will fund, or part-fund, your care home fees. As with England and Wales, your property will be taken into account (as an asset) after the first 12 weeks of residence, in most but not all circumstances.[49] In Northern Ireland social care is more integrated with the health service; there are five health and social care trusts which assess needs.

In **Wales**, most home services involve a charge, up to a maximum of £100 a week. If you have a high income or assets in excess of £24,000 you will mostly have to self-fund. If you have less than £24,000, your income will be considered for the extent of your contribution.[50]

For a place in a care home in Wales, the capital threshold is higher than England's, set at £50,000. If your assets are above £50,000, you will have to self-fund. Below that threshold, you will only have to contribute from income. There will, however, be a limit on how much the local authority will be prepared to pay, so they will inform you which care homes are available that meet your needs within their budget. If you want to stay in a more expensive care home, the local authority may part-fund the residence, while you pay the rest.[51]

Scotland is more generous. As set out above, most home care is free. This applies if you are assessed as needing certain personal care or nursing services. You may, however, have to make a contribution (following a financial assessment) for some home services, such as shopping.[52]

Free personal care and nursing care continues in Scotland when you move to a care home. But other costs, such as accommodation and food, may need to be paid for. They will be assessed on the basis of:

- assets above £35,000: self-funding
- assets below £21,500: state funded (up to £825.94 a week for residential care, 2024–25)
- assets in between the two: part self-funded, part state-funded

You will be assessed on your financial circumstances to decide what, if any, contribution you should make towards costs. As with Wales, if you choose a care home which costs more, you will have to pay the difference.[53]

Now I'll have eine kleine Pause

Kathleen Ferrier (1912–53), last words

Recent History of Reform Proposals

Not surprisingly, there have been many calls for the care system to have a long-term plan. Whether care should be provided by the state at all and, if so, at what cost, has long been controversial.

The Dilnot Commission

Major proposals on funding were made by the Dilnot Commission in 2011.[54] This report is still considered to be the benchmark for care-funding reform. Dilnot's recommendations were framed in the light of the commission's conclusion that the adult care funding system was not then 'fit for purpose'. The key proposals were:

- Responsibility for funding adult social care to be shared between the state and individuals (including those of state pension age)

- A cap on lifetime contributions for care (excluding general living costs), at between £25,000 and £50,000, with £35,000 being 'a fair amount': 'to protect against extreme costs ... and so that people can plan and prepare for the future'
- The asset threshold for paying the full cost of residential care to increase from £23,250 to £100,000
- Unless entirely self-funding, those in residential care should contribute a standard amount towards living costs (eg food and accommodation), such as £7,000 to £10,000 per annum

As to paying for these reforms, Dilnot suggested there were three possible alternatives:

- additional revenue through general taxation
- reprioritising existing expenditure, or
- a specific tax increase (of an existing tax, not a new tax)

Dilnot also recommended that there should be 'more joined-up working across the whole care and support system – health, housing, benefits and adult social care'.

Successive governments have acknowledged that the care system is not as closely integrated with the National Health Service (NHS) as it should be.[55] If you are an older person with a heart problem, the NHS will attend to your needs, free of charge. If you are an older person with dementia, you may have to be of very limited means before you are looked after by the state, in England, at least.

Hospital beds are often not freed up. An elderly patient may no longer need medical care in the hospital, but is not discharged home because arrangements at home for care and support are not in place or a place in a care home is not available. This produces a shortage of hospital beds ('bed-blocking'), delays in A & E departments, logjams of ambulances waiting outside and longer call-out times for ambulances.[56]

Post-Dilnot, The King's Fund (a health and social care charity) berated the lack of government action in reforming the care sector: 'Since 1997 we've had two independent commissions, five White and Green Papers, three consultations and enough reports to fill a library.'[57]

The Health and Social Care Levy

In 2021 the UK Johnson Government proposed a new way to provide increased funding both for the NHS and adult social care for all four nations: a new UK-wide tax, known as the Health and Social Care Levy.[58] This would be funded by an increase of 1.25% in National Insurance contributions (by employers and employees alike) and would provide a £36 billion ring-fenced investment.[59] Further reforms for the UK, including greater integration of the health and social care systems, would be considered in a White Paper.[60]

A cap on personal care

The 2021 proposals also included 'the adult social care *charging reforms*': the introduction of **a cap** of £86,000 on an individual's lifetime spending on personal care (not daily living costs, as in a care home); the increase of the threshold above which a person is not eligible for local authority support (the upper capital limit) from £23,250 to £100,000; and the increase on the lower capital limit from £14,250 to £20,000, with a graduated contribution scheme for a person with assets between £20,000 and £100,000. The template for a cap had been set out in the Care Act 2014, but no cap has been introduced.

But before all this could move forward, the Johnson Government fell (September 2022), and the levy (but not the White Paper) was discarded by the short-lived Truss Government as part of their ill-fated tax-cutting measures (September 2022). The 2021 adult social care charging reforms remained unimplemented.

The Adult Social Care Discharge Fund

A different and more modest plan was, however, announced by the Secretary of State for Health and Social Care in September 2022. The principal focus was to provide 'additional funding ... to help people get out of hospitals and into social care support'. This plan for patients, known as the Adult Social Care Discharge Fund, **was** implemented. Extra money, a relatively modest figure of £500 million, was provided as short-term funding for the ensuing two winters.[61]

Charging reforms delayed

And in November 2022, Chancellor Hunt announced in the Autumn Statement that the charging reforms (above) would be postponed for two years from October 2023 until October 2025. In July 2024, however, Chancellor Reeves, in the new Starmer government, announced that the proposed charging reforms would not be taken forward.[62]

Accordingly, little progress has been made on the core funding for adult social care.

It all goes back to the Dilnot proposals in 2011. Dilnot described the system as 'confusing, unfair and unsustainable'. Unfortunately, nothing of real substance has changed since then in the reform of the care system (except the levy, which was never implemented).

So, despite many recommendations and proposals to make care provision more widely available across the whole of the UK and more integrated with the NHS, reform has repeatedly stalled. There will, no doubt, be change some time, because it is generally agreed that change must come. But when and what remains unclear.

Summary: Some of the Proposals for Change That Have Been Made

		Funding
1	Merge social care with the NHS. Make it free at the point of use. Transfer responsibility (and funding) from local authorities to central government. Increase the overall spending package, from general taxation.	General taxation
2	Make employed people of a certain age, perhaps 40 and over, pay an additional specific tax for social care, ring-fenced funding but limited in the extent of the care to be provided	Specific tax
3	Make those same people (or all working people) liable to pay an additional National Insurance contribution, ring-fenced for social care, with or without contributions from employers	Extra NI contribution
4	Provide a market-based private insurance scheme, with enforced or voluntary contributions	Private insurance contributions

		Funding
5	Keep the mixed state and private provision as now, but place a cap on the contribution that the individual has to pay	General taxation, with capped private contributions
6	Keep the present scheme, but the state to provide specific funding to local authorities for social care	General taxation
7	Increase inheritance tax in order to fund some form of social care	Increased inheritance tax
8	Care pension plan, with those approaching retirement age funding a special pension supported by insurance for extra care needs above a defined threshold	Private funding

CHAPTER 9

Rights

Elderly people have no status. Everybody knows that once you get old and you retire, you don't have any rights as elderly people.[1]

Gwyneth Jones, 77

Older persons, for the purposes of this book and as recognised by the United Nations, the World Health Organisation and the UK Office for National Statistics[2], are adults aged 65 years or over.

They form a substantial and ever-increasing proportion of the United Kingdom population. Nearly 13 million older persons in the UK now fall into this age category, approaching one fifth of the total UK population of about 68.3 million.[3] This is an increase of nearly two million older persons over the last ten years.[4] And this proportion is predicted to increase to one in four by 2050[5].

This, then, is an age group not to be ignored: increasing in size, increasing in working numbers (in good health), increasing in unpaid carer roles, increasing in demands on the health service (in bad health), and increasing, hopefully, in the status of its individuals and the dignity and respect they are afforded.

Why We Need a Charter of Rights for Older Persons

This chapter looks at the growing presence of this older age group and examines their rights. What are the current rights? Are they sufficient? Are they clear? Are they effective?

My conclusion is that more needs to be done. Admittedly, there are rights guaranteed under the Human Rights Act 1998, there are international declarations of principle, and there are specific statutes in the UK such as the Equality Act 2010 which seeks to protect adults from discrimination on the ground of age.

But there is **no single document that defines rights and protections for older persons**. I feel that there is a pressing need for such a document. So I have drafted a Charter of Rights for Older Persons. It would be the first benchmark document of its kind in the UK or in any of the four countries of the UK.

The three essential elements of any charter are:

- the protection of basic rights
- safeguarding the vulnerable
- participation in all decision-making that affects older persons (including national and local policy-making).

Of the three it is the last, perhaps, which has developed the slowest. Giving older persons a voice in everyday decisions which affect them, as well as, through representatives, a voice in national and local policymaking which affects them too, is empowering for this older age group and should be given more thought.

Surely, in the light of history, it is more intelligent to hope rather than to fear, to try rather than not to try. For one thing we know beyond all doubt: Nothing has ever been achieved by the person who says, 'It can't be done.'

Eleanor Roosevelt, one of the authors of the Universal Declaration of Human Rights (1948)

The charter would therefore become a **frame of reference** for all interaction with older persons. From hospitals to care homes, from workplaces to places of recreation, from supermarkets to local shops and cafes, from banks to pension providers, from benefit agencies to council employees – all should have the charter at the forefront of their dealings with older persons. This would lead to basic good practice, based on dignity and respect. All should adopt it and take measures, and where appropriate provide training, to give effect to the charter's objectives.

But first it is necessary to consider what measures exist already.

International Standards

The key, and often repeated, words and phrases in the many internationally respected declarations, conventions and other instruments are:

- dignity
- independence
- equality
- participation
- no discrimination
- no abuse
- care and support services (where necessary)

These are affirmative words, both celebrating the contribution which older persons unquestionably have made to society throughout their lives (and can continue to make) as well as recognising the protection and support that vulnerable older persons undoubtedly need. In 2023, on the UN International Day of Older Persons (1 October), the UN Secretary-General Antonio Guterres referred to older persons as *invaluable sources of knowledge and experience [who] have much to contribute towards peace, sustainable development, and protecting the planet.*

The United Nations (UN) Declaration of Human Rights (1948) was one of the first documents to articulate the fundamental rights that need universal protection. But 1948 was not an age for the rights for older people. The Declaration omits any reference to them.

There is a UN Convention on the Rights of the Child (1989), but no similar convention for older persons.

The UN Principles for Older Persons came much later, in 1991.[6] It notes that individuals in all countries are reaching an advanced age in greater numbers. The UK is not alone in this increase. World numbers of older persons (65 and over) have tripled from 260 million to over 760 million in the last 40 years and are expected to more than double again by 2050.[7]

The UN Principles encourage governments to incorporate for older people the five principles of independence, participation, care, self-fulfilment and dignity into their national programmes whenever possible. But it is no more than exhortation. Governments are not bound to follow it. Wales and Northern Ireland have moved forward to some extent. They both declare that they have regard to the principles and have appointed Commissioners for Older People (**below**). But neither England nor Scotland has a Commissioner.

In addition, the UN has promoted the Madrid International Plan of Action on Ageing (2002). The Madrid Plan acknowledges the contribution of older people to the development of their societies, emphasises the importance of research on age-related issues, and exhorts governments to involve them in socio-economic policy and decision making. Among many other topics, the plan calls for:

- action to be taken to promote employment opportunities for older persons who want to work
- older persons to have greater access to knowledge, education and training
- greater support for older unpaid carers
- solidarity to be fostered between generations, in order to promote social cohesion[8]

The UN Madrid Plan is not, however, legally binding. The implementation of any aspect of the plan by the UK or any government is therefore voluntary.

Some parts of the world have developed their own standards quite separately. They include the Inter-American Convention on Protecting the Human Rights of Older Persons (2015) and the Protocol to the African Charter on Human and Peoples' Rights on the Rights of Older Persons in Africa (2016).

Closer to home, the European Union (EU) has shown a measure of respect for the rights of older people.[9] A European Charter of 'the rights and responsibilities of older people requiring assistance and long-term care' has been proposed, but not implemented.[10] The Charter of Fundamental Rights of the European Union does prohibit discrimination on the ground of age (for age discrimination, *see below*).[11] It recognises and respects the rights of the elderly 'to lead a life of dignity and independence and to participate in social and cultural life'.[12] But nothing more. And, rightly or wrongly, the UK left the EU in 2020, and decided to opt out of the EU Charter[13].

Nevertheless, the Council of Europe (set up after the Second World War)[14] recommended – it cannot dictate – to its 46 member states, including the UK, in 2014, measures for the *Promotion of human rights of older persons*.[15] This aimed, among other things, to raise awareness of public authorities and civic society, so that older persons should be *appropriately consulted, through representative organisations, prior to the adoption of measures that have an impact on the enjoyment of their human rights*. Twenty-one countries responded to the recommendation, not the UK.

Older persons are undoubtedly invaluable. Many persons of this age do not consider themselves 'old'. They live full, active and healthy lives and make considerable contributions to society in many diverse roles and circumstances. Not only are many over 65 in employment or voluntary occupations, but many, estimated to be over ten million in the UK, have a truly significant role as unpaid carers for elderly people and for young grandchildren. Their value is truly invaluable.

The United Kingdom

Back to the UK. In the UK, there is no stand-alone convention, no protocol, no set of principles, no charter. There is no single, coherent, systematic declaratory statement of the rights of older persons.

Even the European Convention on Human Rights (1950), incorporated into our law by the Human Rights Act 1998, makes no claim to provide specific protection for older people. Article 14 of the convention does prohibit discrimination 'on any grounds such as sex, race, colour, language, religion, political or other opinion, national or social origin, association with a national minority, property, birth or other status'. But it makes no mention of discrimination on the ground of age. It is, however, generally considered now that the words 'such as' and 'other status' in article 14 allow the convention to outlaw discrimination also on the ground of age, albeit on a limited basis.[16] And the UK Equality and Human Rights Commission has accepted that the Human Rights Act does not protect against discrimination in all areas of an older person's life (*see below*).

A few local authorities in England, such as Plymouth City Council, the London Borough of Waltham Forest and Thurrock Council, have adopted their own charters, in order to set out what older people can expect from their council and their services. But these are piecemeal and not coordinated

The absence of a national document in the UK on rights for older persons, with protections and participation, speaks for itself. There is clearly a need for a document which sets out a list of minimum standards for older persons.

Ideally, the charter would be incorporated into the law by statute, and be a positive requirement under the law. But for now, it could stand as a **benchmark guideline** for all those who have dealings with older persons. It would be a set of standards against which action and treatment should be measured. It could stand as a yardstick to be followed and respected at all times, and to be an empowering framework for those who are older.

Commissioners for Older People

Some countries have understood the need to represent older people's interests and created special posts of champions for older people, independent of governments. Commissioners have been appointed with responsibility for looking at laws and practices affecting them.

Northern Ireland and Wales both have commissioners. Scotland has had one proposed, but not implemented.[17] England has none.[18] There is a Children's Commissioner in England, but no Commissioner for Older People.

The commissioner in **Northern Ireland**[19], in place since 2011, is directed to *safeguard and promote the interests of older people ... to ensure that Government considers the long-term needs of our ageing population.* Among other things, the commissioner's office provides *advocacy and legal support,* for example to make a complaint about health and social care or about a public authority or about safeguarding or protection or for whistleblowers in care settings.

Wales has had an Older People's Commissioner since 2012.[20] This person is described as *an independent voice and champion for older people across Wales, standing up and speaking out on their behalf.*[21] The commissioner, who is legally obliged to have regard to the UN's Principles for Older Persons:

- takes action in order to protect and promote older people's rights
- takes action to bring an end to ageism and age discrimination
- influences policy and practice at a national and local level
- scrutinises decisions by government and public bodies
- supports older people in Wales with advice and assistance
- listens to what older persons have to say
- sets out the rights of older persons with a Know Your Rights guide

Wales and Northern Ireland set out on their websites[22] some of the rights which are to be promoted. But neither country expresses these rights in a single document. Nor do England and Scotland.

Some other countries have appointed a commissioner or similar role. Australia, for example, has an Age Discrimination Commissioner whose priorities include securing *the wellbeing and safety of older Australians ... to eliminate ageism and age discrimination in Australian workplaces and in the health and social services sectors, improve protection against the abuse of older persons in all its forms.*[23] New Zealand has an Aged Care Commissioner who *advocates for quality health and disability services on behalf of older people.*[24]

In India, the Department of Social Justice and Empowerment has a Senior Citizen Division.[25] Among other things, it funds Elderline, a Nation Helpline for Senior Citizens, and has established a detailed set of Minimum Standards for Senior Citizens' Homes, serving as *a comprehensive guide outlining the benchmarks and criteria essential for the establishment and operation of senior citizens homes across the country.*

In China, there has been a Law on Protection for Rights and Interests of Older Persons since 1996. The Law is designed with a view *to protecting legitimate rights and interests of older persons ... and promoting the Chinese virtue of respecting and supporting older persons.* In 1999 China established a National Commission on Ageing with *the mandate to coordinate and promote ageing-related work access across the country.*[26]

But England has no commissioner. In 2008, England appointed a Voice of Older People, Joan Bakewell (then in her seventies), but the unpaid post lasted only 18 months and has not been filled since. In England there is no Minister and no Commissioner for Older People.

That is not to say that issues relating to older persons are entirely ignored by politicians in Parliament. Certain ministers are responsible for specific topics affecting older people, including adult social care, dementia, mental health, end of life and palliative care, and bereavement. But there is no cohesive approach with a government minister directly responsible for promoting and protecting the interests of older persons.

In 2023 a House of Commons Select Committee[27] launched an important inquiry *on the rights of older persons, examining whether ageist stereotyping and discrimination is preventing them from participating fully in society.* The Women and Equalities Committee chose to inquire into the following topics: digital exclusion, championing older people's rights, intersectionality (requiring distinct policy responses relating to age), stereotyping and discrimination, and labour market access. There is also the less formal All-Party Parliamentary Group (APPG) for *Ageing and Older People*.[28]

As some countries have shown, there is a good case for appointing a person, independent of government, to fulfil the role of commissioner and be a voice, a champion, for issues affecting older people, particularly the issues of health, social care, housing, pensions, benefits, financial hardship, employment and the ever-increasing problem of digital exclusion.

The need for a framework of minimum rights, standards and duties, if not a commissioner, is clear.

Below, then, is my proposed Charter of Rights, for older persons 65 years of age and over.

This Charter establishes a set of **minimum standards for the twenty-first century**. It is a document to be heeded and followed by those who deal with older persons in any context. It is a frame of reference to be observed by partners, close relatives, carers, medical professionals, other professionals (such as solicitors, accountants, bankers), employers, co-workers, activity colleagues, etc. Training should be put in place, particularly for those regularly involved in the employment of or care of older persons.

It is vital, as I have indicated above, that older persons with capacity to do so are involved in decisions which affect them, whether on a daily basis or in the longer term. Others may have their interests at heart, about where to live, how to live, who to live with, but older persons must not be denied their voice. Wherever possible, they need to have the opportunity to lead an independent life in the way they wish.

The voices of older persons also need to be heard in decision-making which affects them at a national and local level, with representatives able to participate in policy-making decisions. Rights for older persons should not only be promoted, they should be discussed and monitored.

A Charter of Rights for Older Persons

1	The right to be treated with respect at all times and to live in dignity
2	The right to be treated fairly and equally
3	The right to independence, self-reliance and autonomy
4	The right to be consulted and to have reasonable wishes respected in decision-making which affects those wishes
5	The right, either directly or through representatives, to have a voice that is heard in national and local policy-making
6	The right to the protection of the law from treatment of a discriminatory, abusive, exploitative or degrading nature
7	The right to a decent and adequate standard of living and as full and normal a life as possible
8	The right to participate in social, cultural and political life, in community life, in appropriate educational and recreational activity, and to have the opportunity to work where possible
9	The right to such care, support and services, including healthcare, social care, housing and community life, as is necessary for wellbeing
10	The right to special care and support where needed, by reason of physical or mental disability or incapacity. And the right, when it is deemed necessary under the law, to curtail rights and movement by reason of mental incapacity, to protection by way of proper legal safeguards, representation and regular reviews.

No document of this kind will be perfect. A charter will have no binding effect in law, unless it is incorporated into statute. But, until then, a breach could be recognised in any claim for discrimination, as a disciplinary offence in the workplace or as the basis for justifiable complaint.

Other Important Rights

Adults of all ages have rights under the law. To some extent they have been protected by the common law of the land over centuries: for example the right of access to the courts[29] and procedural fairness.[30] Or their origin, being derived from elsewhere, may also have been recognised by the courts, such as the right to seek asylum, based on Article 14 of the Universal Declaration of Human Rights (1948).[31]

The Human Rights Act

But the key law for the protection of human rights for all is the Human Rights Act 1998 (HRA). The HRA provides an invaluable protection for all of us in the UK, young and old. It incorporates the European Convention on Human Rights (ECHR) into our law.

The ECHR is an international treaty which could be said to reflect in many respects principles already developed by the common law and other well-known international instruments. It was promoted on our behalf by Winston Churchill MP after the Second World War and was signed by the foreign ministers of the ten founder member European countries in 1949 (Ernest Bevin MP for the UK, the first state to ratify it) as a platform for freedom in Europe.[32]

Thanks to the HRA and the ECHR, we can now rely upon the protection of essential fundamental rights and freedoms. In summary form these are:

- the right to life being protected by law
- the prohibition of torture and inhuman or degrading treatment

- the prohibition of slavery and forced labour
- the right to liberty and security
- the right to a fair trial and no punishment without law
- the right to respect for private and family life, for home and correspondence (the right to privacy)
- freedom of thought, conscience and religion
- freedom of expression and of assembly
- the enjoyment of ECHR rights without discrimination

The HRA protects and enforces these rights by providing each individual with the right to an effective remedy in the UK courts or before the European Court of Human Rights (not to be confused with the European Union's European Court of Justice).

If the UK Parliament were ever to repeal the Human Rights Act, an interesting and essential question would be raised. Would the common law, as developed by the courts, take a step forward in order to protect fundamental rights?

Mental health

There are other rights too, enshrined in Acts of Parliament, which help and support older persons. These include, among others, the right under the Mental Health Act 1983 to healthcare support for mental health and the right under the Mental Capacity Act 2005[33] to participate in decision-making about your life as fully as possible (*see pp 43–51*).

The Mental Health Act 1983, for example, concerns the medical treatment of patients suffering from mental disorder, including the detention of patients and patients' rights. If you are detained ('sectioned'), the Act gives you rights such as the right to certain information, the right to have your views heard, the right to be involved in decision-making, and the right to the assistance of an independent Mental Health Advocate.[34]

The Mental Health Act 2007 amends the 1983 Act. Among other things, it lays emphasis on rights of patients to be recognised and treated as individuals. It provides 'fundamental principles' to inform decisions made under the 1983 Act, including respect for patients' past and present wishes and feelings; involvement of patients in planning, developing and delivering care and treatment appropriate to them; avoidance of unlawful discrimination; and patient wellbeing and safety.

The NHS Constitution

Perhaps the longest list of rights to be aspired to (not fixed in law) is that set out in the little-known NHS Constitution for England (updated 2023). One of the seven 'key principles' is 'The patient will be at the heart of everything the NHS does' (No.4). It includes the words 'Patients, with their families and carers, where appropriate, will be involved and consulted on all decisions about their care and treatment.' It is an NHS 'value' that 'everyone counts': 'We maximise our resources for the benefit of the whole community, and make sure nobody is excluded, discriminated against or left behind.'

The NHS pledges in this constitution, among many laudable objectives, that you have the right:

- to receive care and treatment (free of charge, with exceptions) that is appropriate to you, meets your needs and reflects your preferences
- to be given information about the treatment options available to you
- to accept or refuse treatment that is offered to you
- to be treated with dignity and respect, in accordance with your human rights
- to be protected from abuse, neglect and care and treatment that is degrading
- to privacy and confidentiality
- to access to your own health records and to have any factual inaccuracies corrected
- to be cared for in a clean, safe, secure and suitable environment
- to receive suitable and nutritious food and hydration to sustain health and wellbeing
- to choose your GP practice and to express a preference to be considered for a particular doctor

- to have a complaint you make about NHS services acknowledged within three working days and to have it properly investigated[35]

There are other statutes of relevance in this context. Just by way of example, the Social Services and Wellbeing (Wales) Act 2014 requires care professionals to treat you with dignity and respect; as does Regulation 10 of the Health and Social Care Act 2008 (Regulated Activities) Regulations 2014, for those who are receiving care and treatment from a CQC regulated provider which must also 'support the autonomy, independence and involvement in the community' of their users and have 'due regard' to the protected characteristics (including age) in the Equality Act 2010.

But, high on the list of important rights for older persons, and already mentioned above in various contexts, is protection against **discrimination**, specifically on the ground of age. Ageism and age discrimination should be identified and outlawed at all times. Fortunately, the law against discrimination has developed significantly. Age is now a 'protected characteristic' under the Equality Act 2010, which makes it unlawful to discriminate (directly or indirectly) against a person on the basis of a protected characteristic such as age.

The principle of equality is one of the most fundamental in a democratic society and is certainly one of the most cherished rights of the Convention and the Human Rights Act.[36]

Adath Yisroel Burial Society case (2018)

Age Discrimination

Age is one of the nine 'protected characteristics' under the Equality Act 2010.[37] This means that conduct is unlawful if you are **treated unfairly or harassed on the ground of age**. (The other eight protected characteristics are sex, race, disability, pregnancy or maternity, sexual orientation, religion or belief, or gender reassignment.)[38]

Gradually, albeit slowly, there has been greater recognition of the need for equal treatment for older persons. The old argument that there was no need for special recognition of the elderly because everyone is treated equally, just receiving advantages when they are younger or older, no longer holds sway.

Laws were introduced first to protect older workers[39] and then extended by the Equality Act 2010 (in England, Wales and Scotland). The Act, with a few exceptions, does not apply to Northern Ireland, but there are regulations in Northern Ireland which outlaw employment discrimination on the ground of age.[40]

The Equality Act 2010 can therefore be used to challenge discrimination on the ground of age (or perceived age). In terms of age, discrimination will usually be based on how old you are or the older age group you are in.

The Equality Act applies:

- to the workplace
- to the provision of goods and services
- to the exercise of public functions (**see below**)
- in education
- to associations including private clubs

There are now four main types of age discrimination. They apply particularly in the workplace.[41]:

- **direct discrimination:**[42] treating you less favourably, for example when applying for a job, the employer deliberately favours a younger person, not on ability but on age
- **indirect discrimination:**[43] 'a provision, criterion or practice' that is discriminatory, such as a work practice or protocol or policy which has a disproportionately adverse effect on

older people, putting them at a particular disadvantage, and cannot be justified objectively
- **harassment:**[44] unwanted conduct in relation to age which has the purpose or effect of violating an individual's dignity or creating an intimidating, hostile, degrading, humiliating or offensive environment
- **victimisation:**[45] treating someone badly because they have made (or people think they have made) a complaint about discrimination (such as a whistleblower or any sort of complaint, formal or informal) or have provided information or given evidence in a discrimination case

Since 2012 the law also protects older persons from age discrimination in the provision of goods, facilities and services. The main providers are:

- social services (public or private)
- medical services (GPs, hospitals, dentists)
- transport services
- local authority services
- insurance companies
- shops

It means that you must not be treated less favourably than someone else on the ground of age in any of these contexts, unless an exception applies or good reason can be shown by way of 'objective justification' for the differential treatment.[46]

Goods and services must therefore be provided to older persons in a way which is fair to them. They must, for example, be admitted to a gym or a nightclub, despite being elderly.

If you are considering a complaint or a claim for discrimination against you on the ground of age, the questions which need to be asked are:

- Has there been discrimination? Do you believe you have been treated unfairly or harassed on the ground of age?
- Is the discrimination unlawful? Can it be 'objectively justified'? Is it 'proportionate'?
- Can I bring a claim?

'Objectively justified'

It is not always unlawful to provide a different service based on age. There may be some cases where what would otherwise be age discrimination can be objectively justified, for example, in order to ensure health and safety or protect welfare. Other examples include some financial services, such as insurance companies, which are currently allowed to assess risk based on age. There can also be age-based targeting in health services such as health screening. Holidays can be arranged for certain age groups. Businesses can offer concessions based on age. And free bus passes can be provided for pensioners.

But otherwise, and unless there is some sound reason for different treatment, older people should at all times be treated the same. They should, for example, be charged the same for goods and services as younger people.

'Proportionate'

In some cases, what would otherwise be age discrimination could be lawful because it is a proportionate means of achieving a legitimate aim.[47] A social policy aim which benefits the wider public interest could be proportionate. In 2012, the Supreme Court ruled that a compulsory retirement age of 65 may be proportionate if it has an 'appropriate and necessary' legitimate social policy aim such as staff retention and workplace planning.[48]

By contrast, Employment Tribunals in 2019 and 2023 ruled that Oxford University had unlawfully dismissed active academics on the ground of age. The University had argued, unsuccessfully, that forcing retirement at the age of 68 under their Employer Justified Retirement Age (EJRA) scheme fostered diversity and provided greater opportunities for younger academics. The tribunals found, on the particular facts of each case, that the EJRA scheme was discriminatory in requiring retirement at that age, despite having the legitimate aim of promoting equality and diversity.[49]

(In 2019 the Nobel Chemistry Prize was won by a 97-year-old who had been forcibly retired by Oxford University when he was 65 and had moved to a university in the USA.)

In addition to the Supreme Court case above, cases in the European Court of Justice have referred to policies of inter-generational fairness or for preserving the dignity of older workers as being proportionate.[50] The Equality and Human Rights Commission has also suggested that the following may be proportionate: 'promoting access to employment for younger people' and 'ensuring the mix of generations of staff so as to promote the exchange of experience and new ideas'.[51] Older workers beware.

The Public Sector Equality Duty

The 2012 changes to the Equality Act also prohibited discrimination on the ground of age in the exercise of **public functions** and the running of public clubs and associations. It is a legal requirement for public bodies to avoid direct or indirect discrimination on the ground of age.[52]

Public authorities, such as government departments, local authorities, education bodies, hospital trusts, police, fire and transport authorities, are now required, in carrying out their functions, to have due regard to the need to achieve the objectives in the Equality Act, in particular:

- to eliminate discrimination, harassment and victimization
- to advance equality of opportunity

The Equality and Human Rights Commission has described the purpose of this duty as 'to make sure that public authorities and organisations carrying out public functions think about how they can improve society and promote equality in every aspect of their day-to-day business'. This applies in their decision-making, consideration of policies, providing goods and services and the recruitment, promotion and performance management of employees.

Democracy values everyone equally even if the majority does not.[53]

Baroness Hale of Richmond

Ageism and Discrimination

Ageism is mistreatment of a person by words or action on the basis of age or perceived age. It usually involves one or more of the following: stereotyping, prejudice or discrimination.[54] It can affect any age group. We are concerned here with older people.

Stereotyping involves making generalised assumptions about older people as opposed to treating them individually with their individual differences. Generalised assumptions may involve inclusion of some persons, while excluding others. As an example, 'Older people can't learn new things'; or 'You can't teach an old dog new tricks.'

Prejudice involves negative thinking about older people as a group. For example, 'Older people are better off at the expense of younger people.'

Discrimination involves treating people unfairly because of a characteristic protected under the Equality Act 2010, in this case age (*see p 262*).

The consequences of ageism for the older person may be damaging and hurtful:

- loss of employment or other opportunities
- loss of self-esteem
- exclusion and rejection
- frustration and humiliation
- feeling undervalued
- feeling denied being treated with dignity and respect

Challenging ageism may not be easy. It may be challenged informally, through a word or discussion, making a person or organisation aware at the time or afterwards of their ageist words or action and the resulting consequences. Or it may be challenged more formally, by written complaint, through an organisation's complaints procedure or grievance procedure at work, or, ultimately, in the appropriate tribunal or court.

Taking Action Against Discrimination

Please note that this chapter does not seek to give advice, but merely sets out the basic definitions and some possible alternatives to consider. It is also important to note that a formal claim can be a long process, can be stressful and can be costly. Take advice if you can: from a lawyer experienced in this kind of work, from a trade union if you belong to one, from Citizens Advice or other organisation such as the Equality Advisory & Support Service (EASS) which may be able to help.

The following steps should be considered.

Step 1: Keep a record

In the first place, you should make a full note of what has gone wrong and keep any documentary evidence. Keep a record of dates, times, people (names), places etc. Keep a record of the consequences to you and the effect upon you of the discrimination.

Step 2: Raise your complaint

You should raise your concern (preferably in writing) with the provider of the goods or service, if that is the case, explaining that your complaint is about age discrimination.

If your complaint is against an organisation, there may be a specific complaints procedure.

If your complaint relates to work, first consult your line manager, or, if unsuccessful, use the in-house grievance procedure.

Step 3: Informal resolution

From the start, with any sort of complaint, you should try and avoid any possible misunderstanding, any dispute or the need for a court claim, by seeking informal resolution. Do this by raising your complaint early on with the person or organisation you feel may have discriminated against you.[55]

Informal resolution (including mediation or arbitration) is often the best remedy and may lead to an apology or even a modest offer of compensation. You may wish that some process is put right for others in the future or that staff should receive special training.

Step 4: Formal claim

If all the above fails, and you wish to take your complaint further, write a letter before you enter your formal claim on a claim form. This letter, known as a letter before claim or a letter before action, should set out clearly what claim you intend to make and what it is based on.

In an employment case, there is no need for a letter before claim. Before going to an Employment Tribunal, follow the in-house grievance procedure, then notify the independent Advisory, Conciliation and Arbitration Service (ACAS).

Step 5: County Court or Employment Tribunal

If you wish to make a formal claim on the ground of age discrimination, your claim will, ultimately, be made to:

- the **County Court**, if not related to employment, and should be made within six months of the discrimination;
- an **Employment Tribunal**, if related to work, and should be made (usually) within three months, with notification to ACAS before the claim is made.

Step 6: Proving the claim

Proof of discrimination is not always easy, and often there will be no evidence of direct discrimination. Nevertheless, it is for the employer in a workplace case to prove that there was no discrimination.

There is a risk of costs. The process can be stressful and time-consuming. If you lose your case, you may have to pay the costs of the other party (although that is rare in an Employment Tribunal).

Step 7: A successful claim

If your claim is successful, you will be entitled to **compensation**, the main heads being for:

- loss of earnings
- 'injury to feelings', including stress and anxiety, humiliation, upset (also, where appropriate, psychiatric injury)[56]
- aggravated damages (in very serious cases)

You cannot claim for an apology (although you could have asked for one before the court or tribunal stage).

Employment Tribunals can also make 'appropriate recommendations',[57] for example that staff should undergo special training or that a training policy should be changed.

The Right to Vote

Older people can vote in any election at any age, as long as they are registered on the electoral register.

Older people clearly like to vote. And it is estimated that over 70% of over-75s prefer to exercise their democratic right by voting in person.[58]

That is, perhaps, a little less easy now. The Elections Act 2022 requires voters to produce photo identification with their name matching the electoral register before they can be issued a ballot paper at the polling station.[59] The usual accepted photo ID documents for older persons are a driving licence, passport, older person's travel card or a Blue Badge. Any will do, even if out of date. Or you can apply for a free voting ID card, called a Voter Authority Certificate (or Electoral Identity Card in Northern Ireland), with a recent photo and National Insurance number.[60]

But will this disenfranchise some older persons? Not all will have the requisite ID. They may, for example, no longer have a passport or a driving licence, and, because they have difficulty with forms, are reluctant to apply online or by post for a postal vote. Time, and elections, will tell.

The Right to Die?

There is no right to die, or, at least, not to die early. Euthanasia and assisted dying are currently illegal in the UK. Taking someone else's life deliberately is murder (or, in some limited circumstances, manslaughter). In November 2024 the Terminally Ill Adults (End of Life) Bill, a Private Member's Bill, passed its Second Reading in the House of Commons by 330 votes to 275 and proceeded to further stages of parliamentary scrutiny.

Suicide (taking your own life **and** intending to do so) or attempted suicide has not been a crime since 1961, although encouraging or assisting suicide (helping someone to take their own life) is a crime.[61]

A Society for All Ages

Finally, in the contemplation of rights, one thing should never be forgotten: the contribution that older persons make to life and to the community. Their wisdom, experience and continuing wish to contribute to society are to be treasured. An appreciation of this is expressly stated at the forefront of the UN Principles for Older Persons (1991). It is later repeated in the UN's Madrid International Plan of Action on Ageing (2002), which discerningly encourages the positive fostering of a society for all ages.

CHAPTER 10

After Death

It's not that I'm afraid to die. I just don't want to be there when it happens.

Woody Allen, *Getting Even (1971)*

This chapter reminds you what you need to do *before* you die and advises those you leave behind what they have to do *after* you die. It may sound a little morbid, but it is practical and positive for all.

A Reminder for Those Preparing for the End of Life

There are a number of practical steps for you to take before you die and at a time when you have mental capacity; they're covered in Chapter 1. You should also leave behind your wishes for events after your death (if you want to). In order to help your close family, the following are the key documents to leave behind.

Your Key Documents

1	A will (this is most important)
2	A file containing important information, including • a copy of your will • bank account details • a list of other assets; insurance policies; pension and tax details • contact details for your GP; NHS number • digital access
3	Wishes for burial or cremation
4	Wishes (if any) for the funeral
5	Wishes for disposal of smaller personal items, like pictures and jewellery (if not in your will)
6	Any other reasonable wishes
7	A short history of your life and family (if you wish)

You may think, as you read this, that you won't have to worry about anything after your death. As one correspondent wrote to a newspaper about inheritance tax: 'I won't mind – I will be dead. This will be the optimum moment for me to receive a bill.'[1]

But you can help out. A little planning before death can make all the difference for those who will have to deal with the arrangements after death. It will increase peace of mind for all.

The following are legal and practical steps to be taken after death by those who are left behind.

even the next door
dog stops
barking

Robert MacLean, *Wintermoon (2022)*[2]

For Those Who Will Be Left Behind

When a close member of your family, such as a parent, dies, there are a number of formalities to be complied with. These include:

- registration of the death
- notifying government departments
- burial or cremation
- funeral
- probate

The key important first steps after death are set out below.

For everyone's peace of mind at a difficult time, it will of course help if the formalities and arrangements can be carried out as calmly and efficiently as possible. An agreed plan of things to be done may help. Sensitive compromises may be necessary.

The following table is a summary of the ten steps to be taken, followed by a little more detail on each.

What to Do: The Ten Steps

Early essential steps

1. Obtain the Medical Certificate of Cause of Death (MCCD) from the hospital or your GP
2. Take MCCD to local Registrar of Births and Deaths to register the death
3. Obtain from the Registrar copies of
   - the death certificate (minimum three copies)
   - the 'green form' certificate for burial or cremation and
   - a BD8 certificate about pension and benefits
4. Inform government departments through the *Tell Us Once* service (pension, benefits, tax, driving licence, etc)
5. Instruct a funeral director to make arrangements, including burial or cremation

Further important steps

6. Inform relatives and friends of the death (and funeral arrangements when known)
7. Place notice of death in the press (if required)
8. Plan for the funeral and wake
9. Obtain probate
10. Dispose of small personal possessions

Step 1: Obtain the *Medical Certificate of Cause of Death* (MCCD)

Ask the hospital (if the death was in hospital) or the deceased person's GP (if the death was at home) or, if in a care home or hospice, their GP, to issue the *Medical Certificate of Cause of Death* (MCCD), which will state the medical cause of death. Do this as soon as possible. There is no charge for this document.

The MCCD is sometimes called the 'death certificate' but the Registrar provides another document which is also called the 'death certificate' (*see below*). The MCCD is Form 66.

In effect the MCCD is issued when the doctor is satisfied to the best of their knowledge or belief that the person has died from natural causes. In which case there is no need to report the death to the coroner. The MCCD should record the immediate cause of death and any underlying causes.

Step 2: Register the Death

Take the *Medical Certificate of Cause of Death* (MCCD) and register the death **within five days** (eight days in Scotland) at the Office of Registrar of Births and Deaths, local to where the death occurred: see local authority website for details. You may need to make an appointment.

If to hand, you should take with you to the Registrar:

- the deceased person's NHS card
- birth and marriage certificates
- information (preferably in writing) on:
  - date and place of death
  - proof of full name and last address of person who died (eg a council tax bill)
  - proof of date and place of birth (passport) occupation
  - whether receiving pension or benefits
  - surviving spouse or civil partner's name and date of birth
  - your name and address

Some of the details about the death should be recorded on the MCCD.

Every death must by law be registered with the local Registrar of Births and Deaths.[3] The Registrar will register the death if satisfied that the death was from natural causes.[4] You cannot register the death if it has been referred to the coroner (*see pp 290-291*).

About 580,000 people die in England and Wales every year.[5] Every one of those deaths must be registered (as also in Scotland and Northern Ireland). We have a census every ten years or so to find out who we are, what we do and what we believe in. But we register every single death so that we know who has died, where and when they have died, and what they have died of. It is a full record of deaths and provides learning for the benefit of the health and welfare of the nation.

Step 3: Obtain Documents from the Registrar

- Certified copies of the death certificate as proof of death. Make sure you obtain a number of extra copies (minimum three copies). These are needed for probate, solicitor, banks, insurance companies, pension providers, etc, to prove death.
- The certificate for burial or cremation, known as the 'green form', to be passed to the funeral director (a GRO21 in Northern Ireland).
- A BD8 certificate to send to the Department of Work and Pensions (or use *Tell us Once* service, below) to stop payment of benefits and pension (3344SI in Scotland and 36/BD8 in Northern Ireland).

All forms are free except that there will be a charge for extra copies of the death certificate: currently £11.00 each in England, £8.00 in Northern Ireland, £10.00 in Scotland.

You should also obtain from the Registrar the phone number for the government service *Tell Us Once* and a unique reference number (*see below*).

In Scotland, you will receive, in addition to the Certificate of Registration of Death (to show to the funeral director or the registrar will email it to them,) a shorter copy of the full death entry in the national entry, known as the 'abbreviated' death certificate.[6]

Step 4: Inform Government Departments

Inform government departments of the death. Use the *Tell Us Once* government service: see gov.uk, *Tell Us Once*.

This one-stop service lets you report a death to most government departments in one go.

The *Tell Us Once* service notifies the government departments dealing with:

- pensions
- benefits
- tax and national insurance
- NHS
- driving licences
- passports
- local government services such as disability badge, housing benefit, special services etc.

This service is available in England, Wales and Scotland, but not in Northern Ireland: see nidirect.gov.uk, *Who to tell about a death*.

Step 5: Instruct a Funeral Director

It may be advisable to instruct a funeral director (also known as an undertaker) to make arrangements for burial or cremation, although you do not have to. They will provide invaluable assistance, among a range of services, on booking a religious service or cremation time.

Choose a funeral director service that is local. They will have good local contacts. If you know a local funeral director who has been used by a friend and can be relied on, that may be a good option. If you don't like the funeral director you have chosen, you are entitled to choose another one (although you may have to pay again).

The funeral director should preferably be a member of one of the three trade associations who have Codes of Practice: the National Association of Funeral Directors, the National Federation of Funeral Directors or the Society of Allied and Independent Funeral Directors. There are two large chains: Co-operative Funeral Services and Dignity Funeral Directors. There are also some smaller independent directors. Sometimes the independents may be cheaper.

What does a funeral director do?

A funeral director will discuss with you from the start what services they can provide (and at what cost). There is a wide range of possible services. The key services include:

- taking the deceased person from the place of death (or mortuary) to the funeral director's premises
- preparing the body
- arranging a viewing of the body at the funeral director's chapel of rest (if requested)
- arranging the funeral – time, place, details (in discussion with family members)
- liaising with church, crematorium (and coroner, if necessary (*see below*)
- complying with legal requirements and paperwork
- providing a coffin
- providing transport in cars, limousines or horse-drawn carriage to the funeral
- providing coffin (or pall) bearers

In addition, the funeral director may also provide assistance, if requested, with:

- floral tributes
- programme for the funeral or order of service

- collection of ashes (after a cremation)
- placing an obituary
- arranging a memorial service
- memorial masonry (eg headstone)
- catering for the wake

Fees and costs

Check out the fees in advance. They will include any services you request (as above), including the funeral director's fees, cremation or cemetery fees, the coffin, the hearse and other cars (limousines), flowers and anything else you choose. All of this should be carefully discussed in advance. The average cost of a funeral is rising. It is in the range of £4,000–6,000, but prices vary depending on the services provided and it can cost even more.[7] Burial is more expensive than cremation.

Funeral costs can come out of the person's estate (if there is sufficient money). Some banks and building societies will release funds from the deceased's account to pay for funeral expenses. You will usually need to show the bank a copy of the death certificate and an invoice for the funeral. Otherwise, you will have to wait till the grant of probate before recovering funeral costs from the person's estate.

The **basic costs** usually include mortuary, chapel of rest, coffin, coffin bearers and hearse. Keep an eye out for additional costs. They may include the minister, officiant, burial plot, memorial, limousine hire, death notice, order or service sheets, flowers, catering etc.

If the death was in hospital, the body will be laid out in the hospital mortuary and you will be asked to arrange for the body to be collected by funeral directors. If the death occurs at home or in a care home, you should call the GP immediately. Otherwise you can call an ambulance. Funeral directors will arrange to collect the body and keep in their chapel of rest until burial or cremation.

You do not have to use a funeral director. You can arrange the funeral yourself through your local authority's Cemeteries and Crematorium Department.

Pre-paid funeral plans are payment schemes started in life, a bit like an insurance policy. They allow pre-payment for a funeral. They do not usually cover all the cost of cremation/burial (as often believed), but only a contribution towards them. Funeral costs, it should be remembered, can come out of the deceased's estate.

Some pre-paid funeral plans have been criticised. There have been complaints about mis-selling, unclear terms (such as what is covered in the plan) and unfair charges. And some providers have collapsed financially. Since July 2022, all plan providers are regulated by the Financial Conduct Authority (FCA). Complaints can be made to the Financial Ombudsman Service: see financial-ombudsman.org.uk, *Complaints about pre-paid funeral plans* (updated February 2023).

If you are short of funds, there are charities which may help eg Down to Earth (the Quaker charity).[8] There may be the possibility of a government grant called the Funeral Expenses Payment (sometimes known as a Funeral Payment) by way of contribution towards various costs, including:

- funeral expenses
- burial or cremation fees
- death certificates or other documents
- travel to or from the funeral
- necessary movement of the body over more than 50 miles

You can claim for a Funeral Expenses Payment if you receive certain qualifying benefits and you are the partner of the deceased or a close relative or friend with responsibility for the funeral costs.[9] It should be noted that the government will reclaim this money from any money in the deceased's estate (before any other bills are paid). Make a claim within six months of the death on Form SF200 or call the government Bereavement Service Helpline on 0800 151 2012 for assistance.

Top Five Tips: For Funeral Arrangements

1	Agree on who is to take charge – don't let too many people get involved, although if you need help ask for it, from a trusted family member or friend
2	Be organised: plan and budget (roughly)
3	Let close family know what you are doing: good, clear information always works well
4	Follow the TEN STEPS after death, including respecting the wishes of the person who died
5	It's not about spending money, it's about what feels right, above all for you (and for the person who died)

Moderate lamentation is the right of the dead, excessive grief the enemy to the living.

William Shakespeare, *All's Well that Ends Well* (1601–3)

Step 6: Inform Relatives and Friends

You will need to inform relatives and close friends, particularly those living some distance away, of the death and funeral arrangements (when known) – either immediately or when you feel able.

Compile an email contact list or a WhatsApp group list for notifying relatives and friends of arrangements for funeral and wake. They will want to know as soon as possible, so as to be able to make travel and other arrangements.

Step 7: Place Notice of Death in the Press (If Required)

Put a notice of death in the press, national or local (if you wish to). If the deceased was a well-known person or of special interest, consider an obituary (with photographs).

Step 8: Plan for the Funeral (and Wake)

If there is a will, there may be instructions from the person who died as to their wishes for burial or cremation and the form of the funeral. There may be instructions in an Advance Statement (if there is one, *see pp 30-31*). Although not legally binding, the wishes of the deceased should at least be considered if not followed.

If no wishes have been expressed, it will usually be the responsibility of the partner or nearest relative to plan for the funeral.

Costs are normally recovered out of the estate.

Burial

For a burial or cremation, you need the green form from the Registrar (or the coroner's burial order if the death has been referred to the coroner).

Burials usually take place in a churchyard or in a public or private cemetery,[10] Just by way of example, there are private Muslim cemeteries to the north-east of London run by a (not-for-profit) charity, Gardens of Peace, 'serving the Muslim community in Greater London'.[11]

Burials may also take place on private land (or on a woodland site). Surprisingly, there are few rules about most burials on private land, sometimes home burials. No planning permission or any other special form of consent is required from the local authority or anyone else (although it might be good to let the local authority know, particularly their Environmental Health Department). Consent is, of course, required from the owner of the land and you need to check that there are no restrictive covenants relating to the land which prohibit burial. The Environment Agency[12] does, however, stipulate that there should be at least one metre of soil above and below the body after burial and that the burial should not take place within certain distances of water:

- 10 metres from any 'dry' ditch or field drain
- 30 metres from any spring or any running or standing water
- 50 metres from any well, borehole or spring that supplies water for any use

If there are no relatives or friends to arrange a funeral, the local authority will arrange a simple funeral.

When the Earl of Sandwich died they buried him in between two other guys.

David Carrado[13]

If nobody accepts responsibility for disposal of the body, the state must do so. You do not have to have a funeral. There is no law requiring it.

Cremation

A cremation can only take place at a registered crematorium.[14] There is a crematorium in every part of the country: see local authority website for address.

Cremation is preferred over burial in about 80% of deaths. The first cremation was carried out at Woking, England, on 26 March 1885. Cremations exceeded burials for the first time in 1968.[15]

There are a number of forms for application for a cremation, including Form Cremation 1 (application) and Form Cremation 4 (doctor's medical certificate). Both need to be completed and provided. The funeral director will make these arrangements. These forms and guidance can be found on the gov.uk website under *Cremations taking place in England and Wales: forms and guidance.*[16]

In Scotland, the main form for an adult or child is Form A1.[17] In Northern Ireland, there are just two crematoriums.[18] The cremation forms can be accessed through NIdirect.gov.uk, *Arranging a funeral.*

Cremated ashes can generally be scattered anywhere.[19] Sometimes they are scattered or buried at the crematorium.

Funeral service

A funeral service may be religious but does not have to be. The charity Humanists UK (formerly known as the British Humanist Association) can give advice on a secular service. Other organisations can provide this function too. There does not have to be any service or event at all.

Cremation with a service or event, whether religious or secular, can be held at the crematorium. These services or events vary in style and content. Once I went to a crematorium memorial event where the widow in her eighties sat at the front. She spoke a brief introduction (bravely) and asked anyone who wished to say a few words to do so, rather like a Quaker meeting. They did. It worked very well, especially for her. She was very pleased.

Cremation without a service, sometimes known as 'direct cremation', is a simpler (and usually cheaper) option, without mourners attending. Some sort of ceremony or event can be held elsewhere at a time of your choosing.

Consider whether you want people to give flowers or alternatively make charitable donations. Devise an order of service or event, with a programme of speakers and photographs. What hymns or music? What words or readings? Who should give the eulogy and speak about the deceased person? Who to invite?

Memorial service

Sometimes a later, more public, event is arranged, a memorial service or secular event; it may even just be a memorial party. This sometimes happens when the funeral has been a private family one. The memorial service, arranged for later, will then be open to anyone (or it can be private). It may be advertised in the press or through organisations of which the deceased was a member.

Wake

Plan for the wake (with caterers if required). A funeral director may help you find an appropriate venue.

Consider a budget for all these arrangements. Expenses for funeral directors and other arrangements can come out of the estate of the person who died. Some banks and building societies will release funds from the deceased's account to pay for funeral expenses before probate is granted.

I hope you die before me, because I don't want you singing at my funeral.

Spike Milligan to Harry Secombe

Step 9: Obtain Probate

What is probate?

Probate is the formal legal process whereby the **personal estate** (property, money, possessions) of the person who died is collected and then distributed according to the will (if there is one) or the intestacy rules (if there is not), subject first to the payment of debts and inheritance tax.

Probate is complicated. This section is therefore no more than a summary of the basic legal ground rules. It is based on the law applicable in England and Wales. The rules are similar but not identical in Northern Ireland (see nidirect.gov.uk, *Apply for probate*) and in Scotland where probate is called 'confirmation', a legal document which must be obtained from the Sheriff's Court (see scotcourts.gov.uk, *Dealing with a Deceased's Estate in Scotland*). Different forms apply. In Scotland, there are two types of confirmation: for small estates (valued at £36,000 or less) and for large estates (valued above £36,000).

The process involves:

- locating the most recent will and any codicil(s)
- gathering together the details of the estate's assets and debts (valued as at the date of death)
- calculating whether inheritance tax (IHT) is due: **see Chapter 4**
- paying the IHT (if due) and receiving a code from HMRC
- obtaining a Grant of Probate from the Probate Registry (part of the High Court); this gives formal authority to deal with the estate
- paying the debts of the estate (including funeral expenses, solicitor's fees, mortgages, loans, credit card bills, outstanding utility bills etc)*

- distributing the remaining assets to the beneficiaries
- filing an estate tax return (and paying any income tax or capital gains tax due)

*It may be possible to have funds released *before* the grant of probate in order to pay for reasonable funeral expenses (and the wake) and IHT. The solicitor (*see below*) can apply to banks, insurance companies and other financial institutions for release of funds (if required). They will confirm whether they are prepared to release some funds before probate is granted and, if so, how much.

It is the 'personal representative' who must apply for probate. That person is the **executor**(s) named in the will. A will often names a solicitor as one of the executors and that solicitor will usually be the one who applies for probate. If not, you should choose a solicitor experienced in probate work to obtain probate on behalf of the named executors.

Probate is needed for most estates, but, in broad terms only, it **may not be needed** when:

- the total value of the estate is modest, usually less than £5,000 (subject to individual banks or building societies agreeing to release money without probate)
- the assets of the deceased were not in the deceased's sole name, but were jointly owned (such as a joint bank account or property held by 'joint tenants') and therefore pass to the surviving owner

The probate application form can be completed online[20] or on paper: Form PA1P. There is a fee of £300 if the estate is worth more than £5,000, and £1.50 for each sealed copy.

Probate is complicated. In most cases it is sensible to instruct a solicitor.[21] But you can apply for probate yourself, if you want to, particularly where the estate is uncomplicated. Some people find the paperwork a welcome distraction; others find it challenging.

If a solicitor is instructed, it is very important to clarify the basis of the solicitor's fee before work starts. The fee could be based upon:

- an hourly rate charge

  or
- a fixed (or flat-rate) fee

  or
- a percentage of the value of the estate (to be avoided)

If there is no will, the personal representative will be the next of kin – in order, first the spouse or civil partner, then children over 18, then others listed in the Non-Contentious Probate Rules 1987. That person must apply to the Probate Registry, not for probate, but for a Grant of Letters of Administration in order to be appointed the **administrator** of the estate, fulfilling a similar role to an executor named in a will. Use Form PA1A.

Two key points to underline. If IHT is due, it must (usually) be paid **before** the formal Grant of Probate (or Grant of Letters of Administration) (*see pp 135-137*). And the process of selling a property (which is part of the estate) can be commenced but not completed until **after** the Grant of Probate (or Grant of Letters of Administration).

Step 10: Dispose of Small Personal Possessions

Identify and consider how best to dispose of small possessions. If there is anything of value, it can be sold at auction (or online). The net proceeds of sale belong to the estate. The auctioneer will advise about other possessions of little value. They could go to a charity or be disposed of.

House clearance firms can help, too. They usually charge for removal of possessions, but they may pay you if they think there is enough value in them. Some charities offer this service as well.

If the possessions include documents or small items of family or sentimental value (and no great worth), they can be kept. There should be discussion among close relatives about who should keep them. The person who died may have left wishes about them.

If there are a significant number of possessions of no value at all, such as old clothes not fit for a charity shop, or bedding or old furniture, dispose of them – either at the local tip or through a house clearance firm.

Redirect post through a Post Office (preferably with a copy of the death certificate and your own ID) or online with Royal Mail. There is a Redirection service with Royal Mail for up to 12 months (at a cost) when someone has died (or is subject to a Lasting Power of Attorney). Use the Royal Mail Special Circumstances Redirection application form: see royalmail.com.

Cut down on **junk mail** by registering the death with the Bereavement Register (see thebereavementregister.org.uk) and the Mailing Preference Service (see mpsonline.org.uk), both free services which remove names and addresses from mailing lists. Also contact individual local companies and other organisations to stop their mailings. This can be a slow process.

Benefits

There are a limited number of state benefits available following a death (*see pp 113–114*).

If the death is referred to the CORONER

This section sets out a summary of the legal rules in England and Wales. The rules are very similar in Northern Ireland, although a separate coroner system is in place. Scotland has no coroner system.

The hospital doctor or GP *must* report the death to the local Senior Coroner in a number of circumstances, often when the doctor is not exactly sure of the medical cause of death.[22] In particular, the coroner may become involved where:

- the cause of death is unknown (or the doctor is unsure)
- the death was violent or unnatural or suspicious
- the death may have been due to poisoning
- the death may have been due to an accident or industrial disease or at work
- the death may have been a suicide
- the death occurred in or shortly after being in police or prison custody
- the death may have been due to neglect or self-neglect or in certain medical circumstances such as during some operations

The cause of all deaths in England and Wales which are **not** referred to the local coroner by a doctor are independently double-checked by local Medical Examiners (senior doctors) to make sure that no referral need be made.[23] They are also checked by a Medical Examiner where there is no 'attending practitioner' or none is available within a reasonable time.

There are about 580,000 deaths in England and Wales each year. Around 65% of them are not referred to the coroner.

The other 35% are reported to the coroner. In most of those cases (over 80%) the coroner will make preliminary inquiries (including a post-mortem examination in about 40% of them) and be satisfied that the death was from natural causes and that an inquest is therefore not required. In those cases, the coroner will notify the Registrar that the death can be registered. The doctor will then sign the MCCD which a close family member must take to the Registrar (*see above*).

If the coroner decides to order a post-mortem examination of the body, family members do not have the right to object, but can make their wishes or those of the deceased (particularly religious wishes) known to the coroner before the examination is carried out.

Only in about 15% of deaths referred to the coroner will the coroner take the investigation to an inquest (although this is still 37,000 inquests a year, under 500 with a jury). The coroner must do so where s/he has 'reason to suspect' one of the following:

- the deceased died a violent or unnatural death
- the cause of death is unknown, or
- the deceased died while in custody or otherwise in state detention

Where the death is reported to the coroner, a close family member cannot register it until the coroner gives permission, either where no inquest is required or after the inquest if one is held.

If there is to be an inquest, the coroner can provide a close family member with an interim death certificate as proof of death (also sometimes known as a death certificate). You can use this document as proof of death when you inform banks and other organisations and when you apply for probate.

If there is an inquest, with or without a jury, the inquest will provide:

- the answers to the four statutory questions: who died, how, when and where did they come by their death
- the medical cause of death
- a conclusion as to the death

These answers will be set out in the Record of Inquest, a public document which should be kept by the local coroner's office for all time.

Top Ten Tips

1	**Make a plan**, a list for everything that has to be done – there is much more to do than some might expect	
2	Follow the first **5 ESSENTIAL STEPS** immediately	1. Obtain MCCD 2. Register the death 3. Obtain documents from Registrar 4. Inform Government departments 5. Instruct funeral director
3	Follow the **FURTHER 5 STEPS**	6. Inform relatives/friends 7. Notice of death 8. Plan for funeral 9. Obtain probate 10. Arrange disposal of personal possessions
4	**Follow the wishes of deceased** where possible (for example on organ donation, burial or cremation, nature of funeral). The wishes may have been told to you in person or set out in a will or Advance Statement (*see pp 13, 30*). In law, you do not have to follow the deceased's wishes.	
5	**Consider the wishes of others**, for example on the funeral and wake. Discuss and agree where possible, but don't be overwhelmed by other people's wishes or demands if it is your responsibility to make arrangements.	
6	**Obtain probate** (through a solicitor or do it yourself). This is usually the last of all necessary legal steps and therefore may bring some element of closure.	
7	**Consider whether inheritance tax may have to be paid** – this is part of the probate process (*see pp 135–137*)	

8	If the death is referred to the coroner, **keep in touch with the coroner's officer**. If there is an inquest, you may be entitled to copies of documents (if you wish to see them), eg the post-mortem report and witness statements.
9	Many people like to **make a memory box** or file with treasured memories, photos, certificates of birth and marriage, short history (*see pp 41–42*). It can help to celebrate and continue to celebrate a life.
10	**Look after yourself, physically and mentally** – this is a difficult and demanding time. Take bereavement counselling, if appropriate.

Afterword

There is always so much to do, and at a time of loss. I hope this last chapter eases some of the burden.

I hope, too, that for all of us over 65, or those of you of a younger age who are thinking towards your own later years or the later years of others who may need help, this book provides some useful pointers in the right direction. Or, at least, has given you pause for thought. What you choose to do and how you do it is, of course, entirely up to you. Whatever that is, I wish you well with it. I hope it brings a little peace of mind for your well-earned later years.

Appendix

*The following is an illustration of an **Advance Decision** (pp 19-29) together with an **Advance Statement** (pp 30-31). You can choose to write either or both. Only the Advance Decision is legally binding and only if it is in the proper form. There is no dedicated form for either document.*[1]

The Wishes of [Name]: **Advance Decision** and **Advance Statement**

An example

These are the wishes of:

NAME ....

ADDRESS ....

DATE OF BIRTH ....

NEXT OF KIN ....

GP – NAME, ADDRESS, TELEPHONE NUMBER

NHS NUMBER ....

Introduction

[*Notes for assistance are set out in italics. They should not become part of the text.*]

1. These are my wishes concerning end of life medical care (Advance Decision) and other decisions (Advance Statement) in the event of my suffering mental incapacity within the meaning of the Mental Capacity Act 2005. They are also my wishes on death.

2. Unless and until I lose mental capacity, please do not treat me medically without consulting me and considering my wishes. If I become physically disabled but of sufficient sound mind so as to be capable of making informed decisions within the meaning of the Mental Capacity Act 2005, allow me to make decisions about care and end of life.

3. I currently have mental capacity for the purposes of the Mental Capacity Act 2005. I am 68 years of age and I am still working (part-time). I work as a . . . and as a . . . Both these jobs

require accounting skills. I also volunteer for a charity where I teach English as a foreign language to immigrants on work visas.

OR

I have been assessed by my GP, Dr . . . as having mental capacity in accordance with the Mental Capacity Act 2005 for the purposes of making this document. Dr . . .'s assessment is attached to this document. [*OR* Dr . . . has signed this document to acknowledge that I have mental capacity.]

4   I have also made Lasting Powers of Attorney (LPAs) for both (a) health and welfare and (b) property and financial affairs. They are registered LPAs Nos. XX and XY, dated [*add DATE*] respectively. My attorney(s) is/are [*NAME, CONTACT DETAILS*].

Advance Decision

5   This part of my wishes is my Advance Decision. I make it to express my wishes for refusing medical treatment in specific circumstances. [My GP (above) has a copy of this Advance Decision.]

6   I intend this document to apply even if my life is at risk. [*This sentence must be included if this document is to be legally binding.*]

7   I believe I currently have mental capacity for the reasons set out in paragraph 3 above. [My GP has signed this document to acknowledge that I have mental capacity.] I do, however, recognise that there may come a time, whether from stroke or dementia or brain damage or other illness or injury, that I will be assessed to lack mental capacity. It is with regard to these possible circumstances in the future that I write this Advance Decision document. I have carefully considered these decisions.

8 I make this Advance Decision of my own free will.

9 **I wish to refuse all life-sustaining treatment** when offered by healthcare professionals in the event that I am suffering from:

   a diseases of the central nervous system, including but not limited to motor neurone disease, Parkinson's Disease and Huntington's Disease
   b brain injury, including but not limited to stroke, vegetative or minimally conscious states
   c any form of dementia including Alzheimer's disease
   d any terminal illness or
   e other [*specify*] [*It is your choice which you include.*]

   Do not attempt to resuscitate me in any of these circumstances.

10 For the purposes of this Advance Decision **I refuse all life-sustaining treatment** in these circumstances, including but not limited to **the following treatment:**

   - cardiopulmonary resuscitation (CPR) in the event that I stop breathing or my heart has stopped beating, whether by chest compressions, electrical shocks or otherwise, particularly (but not limited to) in a potential end-of-life medical situation
   - artificial ventilation
   - artificial nutrition and hydration (ANH)
   - antibiotics
   - chemotherapy
   - organ transplant
   - kidney dialysis

   [*You may choose any one or more or all of these different treatments.*]

11 [*In addition to the above circumstances you may wish to add* **one or more** *of the following circumstances. This will further limit your intention to refuse treatment.*]

I refuse all life-sustaining treatment in the circumstances above, but only when I am:

- oblivious of my surroundings
- unable to recognise close family or friends
- constantly agitated or distressed, or
- incapable of caring for my own hygiene

12 I wish this Advance Decision on refusing life-sustaining treatment to override the authority of the attorney(s) under the existing or any future Lasting Power of Attorney in this respect. [*If you have made or may in the future make a health and welfare LPA.*]

13 My reasons for this Advance Decision are that I do not wish to have my life prolonged in a way or at a time:

- when the quality of my life has become or will become poor or poorer
- when I may be further disabled by attempts at resuscitation, or
- when there is a real possibility of continuing or increased pain and suffering

I wish to avoid grievous end-of-life suffering for myself and for those who will have to witness it, namely my partner, children, close relatives and close friends.

[*This paragraph is not legally required, but you may wish to consider it.*]

14 In the above circumstances I wish to receive palliative care where appropriate, including treatment to make me comfortable, such as pain relief.

[*You are not allowed by law to refuse this kind of treatment anyway. But you may wish to assert this wish.*]

Advance Statement

15 In addition to my Advance Decision above, I wish to set out in this Advance Statement my wishes for the future in the event of losing mental capacity. I understand that these wishes are not legally binding, but I would like family, carers and healthcare professionals to take account of them in their dealings with me.[2]

Care

16 I wish to stay in my own home as long as is feasible and to be cared for by professional carers who shall be paid for out of my own funds. I would prefer carers to visit rather than live in.

OR

If I lose mental capacity, I wish to be cared for at the discretion of the State. I have limited funds and am unable to pay for my own care.

17 I wish the following to be consulted about my care: my partner (if surviving) and my eldest child. [*Name them. Others can be named, as you wish.*]

Beliefs

18 My religion is Roman Catholic. I am not a practising churchgoer but wish if possible to be attended upon and receive communion and when appropriate the last rites from a priest.

OR

19 I am an atheist/non-believer and request respect for this belief (or lack of it). For example, I do not wish to be visited by priests or vicars in the last days of life.

Personal

20 I wish to be called by the name 'Jim'. James is my middle name, not my first name, but I have always been known as 'Jim'.

21 I like tea first thing in the morning (and at teatime) and coffee mid-morning.

22 As a hot meal I always prefer chicken, but I like fish too. I like fresh vegetables, and soups and salads.

23 If I am no longer able to go to (or be taken to) the pub for a pint of beer, my alcoholic drink of choice is red wine.

24 I like dramas and thrillers on TV. I listen to the radio a lot and especially news and current affairs programmes.

25 I prefer a shower to a bath.

26 I do not like to be fussed about. I am a straightforward Lancastrian (and probably a bit obstinate).

On death

27 On death, as an organ donor on the NHS Organ Donation Register[3], I wish any useful organ or tissue to be retained and, where possible, used for the medical benefit of another or others.

28 Subject to organ and tissue donation, I wish to be cremated with a brief religious ceremony conducted by a Catholic priest at the crematorium.

OR

29 Subject to organ and tissue donation, I wish to be cremated with a non-religious ceremony.

OR

30 Following a Catholic funeral service at St Hilda's, I wish to be buried in the cemetery there.

31 I would like my partner (if she survives me), or my eldest child (if she does not), to organise the order of service. I would like the music to include something from Vivaldi's Four Seasons. I would like the hymns Abide With Me and Praise To the Lord the Almighty. I would like my brother George to speak about me (if he feels able). I would like there to be a reading from the bible, such as Psalm 23.

32 If anyone wishes to write an obituary about me, I wish it to include some reference to my keeping wicket for the ABC Cricket Club for 20 years.

33 I would like the wake, if there are sufficient funds, to be held in the pavilion of the ABC Cricket Club.

SIGNED by me ....
DATED ....
WITNESSED by ....
Name ....
Relative/friend ....
DATED ....

Updated

I confirm that the above document sets out my present wishes.

SIGNED by me ....
DATED ....

Notes

Introduction

1. A number of life insurance companies have surveys to that effect, including, for example, Canada Life UK, March 2023: more than half of all adults, and one third of the over 55s, have not made a will.
2. Office for National Statistics (ONS), *Overview of the UK population: August 2019* (August 2019). See also House of Commons Library, *The UK's changing population* (July 2024); Office for National Statistics (ONS), *Population estimates for the UK, England and Wales, Scotland and Northern Ireland: mid-2023* (October 2024); The Institute for Fiscal Studies (IFS), *UK health and social care spending* (February 2017). And worldwide, the population of persons aged 65 and over, some 761 million in 2021, is expected to more than double, to 1.6 billion, in 2050: UN, Department of Economic and Social Affairs, *Leaving No One Behind In An Ageing World* (World Social Report 2023). See also World Health Organisation (WHO), *Ageing and health* (October 2021).
3. ONS, *Estimates of the very old, including centenarians, England and Wales: 2002 to 2023* (October 2024): 15,152 in 2022, more than double than in 2002, and more than four times as many women than men.
4. Apologies if any of these distinguished persons have since died. For consistency, I have omitted their various titles.
5. NHS England *Improving care for older people*, citing Barnett et al., 2012.
6. See gov.uk, *Check your State Pension age*. The pension age was equalised for men and women (at age 65) in November 2018.
7. UN, Department of Economic and Social Affairs, *Leaving No One Behind In An Ageing World* (World Social Report 2023). WHO, *Promoting physical activity and healthy diets for healthy ageing in the WHO European Region* (October 2023). NHS England, *Improving care for older people*. ONS, *Living longer: Is the age of 70 the new age 65?* (November 2019): 65 is 'the traditional age as the marker for the start of older age'. 65 is also the age for EU statistical purposes: Eurostat. Some academics have suggested that an older age should be set: see, for example, *Redefining the elderly as aged 75 years and older: Proposal from the Joint Committee of Japan Gerontological Society and the Japan Geriatrics Society* (July 2017).
8. Penguin, 1963.
9. The Friendly Societies Act 1875, section 8(1).
10. See Note 7.

CHAPTER 1
Before Death

1. Seneca, *How to Die* (Princeton University Press, 2018).
2. See Law Society of Scotland, *Making a will*.
3. See, for example, the Law Society's helpful *Elderly Client Handbook* (6th Edn., 2019), pp 17–19.
4. For further information, see the (not-for-profit) Digital Legacy Association at digitallegacyassociation.org.
5. See facebook.com, *Managing a deceased person's account*; instagram.com, *Memorialise or close a deceased person's Instagram account*; paypal.com, *How do I close the PayPal account of a deceased relative?*
6. See gov.uk, *Search probate records for documents and wills (England and Wales)*. See also House of Commons Library, *Obtaining a copy of a will* (October 2022).
7. A caveat is a formal objection to the validity of a will, by way of challenging someone else's application for probate. See gov.uk, *Stopping a probate application*: Apply for a caveat online or by post; the cost is currently £3.
8. Under the Inheritance (Provision for Family and Dependants) Act 1975.
9. See gov.uk, *How to store a will with HM Courts and Tribunals Service (HMCTS)* (updated May 2024). The fee is currently £20. Use envelope label PA7ENV. For assistance phone the probate helpline on 0300 303 6048.
10. For further information see, for example, Age UK, Factsheet 72, *Advance decisions, advance statements and living wills* (April 2024); Alzheimer's Society, *Dementia, advance decisions and advance statements*; Compassion in Dying, *Make an advance decision (living will)*; Macmillan Cancer Support, *Advance decision to refuse treatment*. According to the charity Compassion in Dying, only 4% of the population have made an Advance Decision, despite 82% having strong views about end-of-life treatment (January 2016); 2% in Wales: Wales Centre for Public Policy, *Increasing Understanding and Uptake of Advance Decisions to Reform Treatment in Wales* (February 2016).
11. Advance decisions to refuse treatment (ADRTs) are governed by Sections 24–6 of the Mental Capacity Act 2005.
12. See gov.uk, *Mental Capacity Act Code of Practice* (updated 2020), Chapter 9.
13. See gov.uk, *Mental Capacity Act Code of Practice* (updated 2020), Chapter 9.
14. See information for patients and those close to them provided by the medical charity, the Resuscitation Council UK at resus.org.uk: *Decisions about Cardiopulmonary Resuscitation (CPR); Guidance: CPR;* and *CPR Recommendations, DNACPR and ReSPECT*.
15. See digital.nhs.uk, *How NHS Digital is helping improve cardiac arrest outcomes* (October 2021). See also lower figures, eg 7–8% for out-of-hospital cardiac arrests: (OHCA, 2024) (30,000 each year); england.nhs.uk, *Resuscitation to Recovery* (March 2017); and National Institute for Health and Care Excellence (NICE, September 2023); 10.8%, londonambulance.nhs.uk, *We release new stats on cardiac arrests showing survival rates outside of hospital reach all time high* (January 2020); 12% for OHCAs; cf. a higher figure of 24–40% for in-hospital arrests, bmj.com, *Patients Overestimate the success of CPR* (July 2020).
16. See gov.uk, *Mental Capacity Act Code of Practice* (updated 2020), paragraph 9.28.

17 Section 2, Suicide Act 1961.
18 For an example of an Advance Decision being tested, see *Re PW (Jehovah's Witness: Validity of Advance Decision)*, [2021] EWCOP 52. The English court held that (1) if an advance decision to refuse a blood transfusion were held to be valid, it had to be respected even though it might lead to death; (2) if it were not valid and the person lacked capacity at the time to make the decision, the question to be asked would be What decision should be made on her behalf in her best interests?
19 See T Meek, A Ruck Keene et al., Association of Anaesthetists, *Implementing advance care plans in the peri-operative period, including plans for cardiopulmonary resuscitation: Association of Anaesthetists clinical practice guidance* (February 2022).
20 See the Recommended Summary Plan for Emergency Care and Treatment (ReSPECT) on the Resuscitation Council website. See also joint guidance from the BMA, Resuscitation Council (UK) and Royal College of Nursing: BMA, *Decisions relating to CPR (cardiopulmonary resuscitation)* (updated August 2021); NHS England and nhs.uk, *Do not attempt cardiopulmonary resuscitation (DNACPR) decisions*.
21 Section 4(1), Adults with Incapacity (Scotland) Act 2000. See also Scottish Government, *Do Not Attempt Cardiopulmonary Resuscitation (DNACPR) – integrated adult policy: guidance* (May 2010).
22 See Solicitors for Older People Scotland, *Guide to Advance Directives* (August 2016); Macmillan Cancer Support, *Advance Directive*.
23 The relevant sections of the Mental Capacity (Northern Ireland) Act 2016 are not yet in force.
24 See the Department of Health's *Review of the Law Relating to Advance Decisions to Refuse Treatment* (June 2019).
25 See, for example, Department of Health, Northern Ireland, *Advance Care Planning Policy for Adults in Northern Ireland, Draft Policy for Public Consultation* (December 2021).
26 For further information on Advance Statements, see Note 10.
27 See section 4(6)(a), Mental Capacity Act 2005.
28 See sections 275, 276, Mental Health (Care and Treatment) (Scotland) Act 2003, as amended by the Mental Health (Scotland) Act 2015.
29 See nhs.uk, *Advance decision to refuse treatment (living will)* and *Advance statement about your care wishes*; Financial Ombudsman Service, *Power of Attorney* (updated January 2021).
30 Separate arrangements exist for Scotland and Northern Ireland.
31 Information from the Office of the Public Guardian (OPG), 2017–18. See also the OPG *Annual report and accounts 2022–23* (September 2023).
32 The Enduring Powers of Attorney Act 1985 was replaced by the Mental Capacity Act 2005, with Lasting Powers of Attorney introduced in 2007.
33 See gov.uk, *Lasting power of attorney forms* (updated April 2024).
34 In order to protect against fraud and abuse, the Powers of Attorney Act 2023 also creates new ID checks on those applying for an LPA.
35 See gov.uk, *Make, register or end a lasting power of attorney*. Over one million applications are made each year. There are more than 6 million LPAs in existence.
36 See the Lasting Powers of Attorney, Enduring Powers of Attorney and Public Guardian Regulations 2007.

37 See gov.uk, *LPA and EPA fees, LPA120*.
38 See gov.uk, *Make, register or end a lasting power of attorney*. See also gov.uk, Office of the Public Guardian, *About our services* (November 2024) which states: 'Allow up to 16 weeks ... [for] your LPA ... application to be processed.'
39 See gov.uk, *Use a lasting power of attorney*.
40 Section 1, Powers of Attorney Act 1971 (as amended by the Powers of Attorney Act 2023).
41 See sections 15–24, Adults with Incapacity (Scotland) Act 2000. See Office of the Public Guardian (Scotland), *What is a power of attorney?*
42 For a template, see The Law Society of Northern Ireland, *EPA – Enduring Power of Attorney Form*, as prescribed by the Enduring Power of Attorney Regulations (NI) 1989. See also the Enduring Power of Attorney (Northern Ireland) Order 1987.
43 See Department of Justice (Northern Ireland), *Information on Enduring Powers of Attorney (EPA)*. See also nidirect.gov.uk, *Managing your affairs and enduring power of attorney*.
44 See, for example, autodotbiography.com; storyvault.com; mylifestorybook.com; boundbiographies.com. See also the self-help book, *Writing Your Autobiography*, Jackie Sherman (Emerald Publishing, 2011).
45 Cited by Muriel Spark in *Loitering with Intent* (Virago Modern Classics, 2007).
46 The concept of *mental capacity* (in England and Wales) is governed by the provisions of the Mental Capacity Act 2005. See also gov.uk, *Mental Capacity Act Code of Practice* (updated October 2020), issued under sections 42, 43 of the MHA 2005. Much helpful guidance on mental capacity and the 2005 Act is provided by the NHS at nhs.uk, the General Medical Council at gmc-uk.org, the Care Quality Commission at cqc.org.uk, and by various charities on their websites, such as Carers UK, the Mental Health Foundation, Mind and Marie Curie. Alex Ruck Keene KC (Hon), Visiting Professor, King's College London, provides helpful advice and discussion in his blog mentalcapacitylawandpolicy.org.uk. See also Jonathan Herring, *Vulnerable Adults* (OUP, 2009).
47 Section 1(2), Mental Capacity Act 2005 (MCA 2005).
48 For Scotland see the Adults with Incapacity (Scotland) Act 2000. For Northern Ireland see the Mental Capacity (Northern Ireland) Act 2016 (not yet in force).
49 Section 5(1), Mental Capacity Act 2005.
50 Section 5(1), Mental Capacity Act 2005.
51 See the helpful BMA, *Mental Capacity in Northern Ireland* (updated March 2024); BMA, *Adults with Incapacity in Scotland* (updated January 2024). See also Note 48.
52 *Re MB* [1997] EWCA Civ 3093.
53 Section 1(6), Adults with Incapacity (Scotland) Act 2000. See also the helpful summary at Carers.uk, *What is mental capacity?* See also guidance provided by the Scottish Government in a number of documents including gov.scot, *Social Care, Adults with Incapacity*; and the Office of the Public Guardian (Scotland), *Adults with Incapacity (Scotland) Act 2000*.
54 Section 1(2), Adults with Incapacity (Scotland) Act 2000.
55 Section 1(6), Mental Capacity Act 2005.

56 Section 4(2), Mental Capacity Act 2005.
57 Section 4(6)(a), Mental Capacity Act 2005.
58 See Alex Ruck Keene KC's blog at Note 46.
59 The Mental Capacity (Amendment) Act 2019. The proposals for LPS came on the recommendation of the Law Commission: Law Commission, *Mental Capacity and Deprivation of Liberty* (No.372, March 2017).
60 Sara Gruen, *Water for Elephants* (Allen & Unwin, Algonquin Books, 2007).

CHAPTER 2
Money

1 Institute for Fiscal Studies: Report by Jonathan Cribb, Agnes Norris, Keiler, Tom Waters, June 2018 – *Living Standards, Poverty and Equality in the UK: 2018* and *2024* (see ifs.org.uk).
2 Tracey Crouch, Minister for Sport and Civil Society (January 2018). Under the Dormant Assets Scheme (see the Dormant Assets Act 2022), over £1.5 billion has been transferred into the scheme, with £800 million released for charitable purposes. See gov.uk, *Dormant Assets Scheme: statement of intent overview* (September 2023); Reclaim Fund Limited, a not-for-profit organisation, at reclaimfund.co.uk.
3 See *Which? How investment platforms work* (April 2024).
4 MoneyHelper (the government-supported independent website) and other websites have their own budget planners or templates and provide money management advice. Or you can buy a ready-made budget planner.
5 Popularised by US Senator Elizabeth Warren.
6 *FTMoney* (December 2018).
7 See moneyhelper.org.uk, *Choosing a financial adviser* and *Key questions to ask your financial adviser*; unbiased.co.uk, *How to choose the right financial adviser in the UK* (updated October 2024); citizensadvice.org.uk, *Getting financial advice*.
8 Office for National Statistics, *People aged 65 years and over in employment, UK: January to March 2022 to April to June 2022* (September 2022); Rest Less, *The number of over 70s still working has more than doubled in a decade to nearly half a million in 2019* (May 2019, pre-pandemic); Rest Less, *Number of men aged 70 plus in work has increased by 58% in ten years* (May 2023).
9 ONS, *Labour market overview, UK: August 2024* (August 2024).
10 See restless.co.uk, *Top 15 part-time jobs for the over 50s* (April 2024).
11 A study of 8,700 people in their 50s and older by Northwestern University and University of Michigan, published in the *Journal of the American Medical Association* (April 2018).
12 Alan Garber, Professor of Health Policy at Harvard University, commenting on the above.
13 John Lanchester, *London Review of Books* (5 July 2018).
14 For 2024/25. Increased from £15,240 in 2016/17.
15 See gov.uk, *Commentary for annual savings statistics: September 2024* (November 2024).
16 The Lifetime ISA (LISA) must be opened before you are 40, although further payments, up to £4,000 pa, can be made into it until the age of 50. The LISA replaced the Help to Buy ISA in 2019.

17 moneyhelper.org.uk, *What is equity release?*
18 See MoneySavingExpert, *Should you equity-release?* (updated August 2024).
19 See MoneySavingExpert, *How to check your credit report for free* (updated September 2024).
20 Try, for example, comparethemarket.com, confused.com, GoCompare, MoneySuperMarket and Quotezone (for car insurance). See also, Laura Whately, *Money: A User's Guide* (Fourth Estate, 2020): one of her ten 'surprising' ways to save money is *Never be Faithful*.
21 currentaccountswitch.co.uk claims that over 10 million current account holders have used the service and more than 50 banks and building societies participate.
22 Citizens Advice, *The insurance loyalty penalty: unfair pricing in the home insurance market* (November 2017).
23 Financial Conduct Authority, *FCA confirms measures to protect customers from the loyalty penalty in home and motor insurance markets* (May 2021), bringing pricing, auto-renewal and data reporting rules into effect on 1 January 2022.
24 Loyalty penalties in these markets total £1.3 billion pa: see Citizens Advice, *One-in-seven customers still paying the loyalty penalty despite cost-of-living crisis* (August 2022). Regulators do not always find it easy to bring service providers into line for the benefit of the customer. For example, Ofcom announced in September 2021 that *One Touch Switch*, a new set of rules to make it easier to switch your broadband provider without having to notify your current provider, would come into force in April 2023. But that same month Ofcom was forced to open 'an industry-wide enforcement programme' because of 'failed implementation' by broadband providers.
25 University of Nottingham, with Browne Jacobsen, solicitors (2018).
26 See energysavingtrust.org.uk, *Quick tips to save energy* (updated November 2024); *Top ten energy saving tips*.
27 See gov.uk, *HMRC interest rates for late and early payments* (updated August 2024). For example, the interest rates from 20 August 2024 are 7.5% for late payment, and 4% for repayment.
28 See gov.uk, *How to pay a debt to HMRC with a Time to Pay Arrangement* (updated November 2021).
29 See moneyexpert.com, quoting *Which?* (November 2018). Since 2015, 6,161 branches of banks and building societies have closed, ie about 53 on average per month: *Which?, Bank branch closures: is your local bank closing?* (September 2024). And not everyone has a bank account; 1.1 million have no current account and are 'unbanked': FCA, *Financial Lives 2022 Survey* (updated March 2024).
30 Financial Conduct Authority (FCA), *FCA sets out new rules to maintain access to cash in increasingly digital world* (December 2023). See also, ukfinance.org.uk, *UK Payment Markets Summary 2022 (August 2022);* and Age UK, *How the decline of cash is affecting older people* (June 2021).
31 UK Finance, *UK Payment Markets 2024* (July 2024). See also British Retail Consortium, *Payments Survey 2023* (December 2023).
32 According to LINK, the UK's largest cash machine network, a not-for-profit organisation: see link.co.uk, *Data & Research* (April 2024).
33 Section 54 and Schedule 8 of the Financial Services and Markets Act 2023, amending the Financial Services and Markets Act 2000; gov.uk, Policy paper, *Cash Access Policy Statement* (August 2023).

34 See FCA, Note 30. One of the purposes of the policy was to avoid the provision of access to cash services declining in 'a disorderly way'.
35 For more details, see MoneySavingExpert, *Section 75 refunds* (updated August 2024).
36 The Money Charity, *The Money Statistics September 2024*.
37 Financial Conduct Authority, *FCA tells credit card firms to review their approach to persistent debt customers* (February 2020).
38 See also Money Advice Trust, 'a national charity helping people across the UK to tackle debts and manage their money with confidence'.
39 49.7% in 2021, 49.4% in 2022: see ONS, *Population estimates by marital status and living arrangements, England and Wales: 2022* (January 2024).
40 See House of Commons Library, *'Common law marriage' and cohabitation*, 22% (November 2022); Office for National Statistics, *People's living arrangements in England and Wales: Census 2021*, 24.3% (February 2023).
41 See The Law Society, *Moving in together: getting a cohabitation agreement*; *Cohabitation – your rights*.
42 See generally, Citizens Advice, *Living together and marriage – legal differences* and *Living together, marriage and civil partnership*.
43 See Helen Dewdney's excellent books *How to Complain* (The Complaining Cow, 3rd Edn. 2015, updated 2019), and *101 Habits of an Effective Complainer* (2019). See also her website www.thecomplainingcow.co.uk and her *Top 20 Tips for How to Complain Effectively*
44 See financial-ombudsman.org.uk, *Annual complaints data and insight 2023/24* (July 2024).
45 See financial-ombudsman.org.uk, *Compensation* (April 2024), for complaints from 1 April 2024.
46 See Financial Conduct Authority, *Consumer Duty implementation: good practice and areas for improvement* (updated February 2024).
47 Updated March 2024.
48 Updated May 2023.
49 *The Sea, The Sea*, by Iris Murdoch (Chatto & Windus, 1978).

CHAPTER 3

Pensions and Pension Credit

1 The Pensions Act 2011.
2 The Pensions Act 2014 (changing the projected pension age in the Pensions Act 2007 of 67 from 2034–36). See also gov.uk, *State Pension age review 2017* (updated July 2017) and *State Pension age Review 2023* (March 2023).
3 See The Pensions Act 2007. In 2017 the government accepted the recommendation of the first Review of State Pension age that the rise to 68 should be in 2037–39, but the Department for Work and Pensions, Policy paper, *State Pension age Review 2023* (March 2023) was less certain and deferred the decision as to when that increase should be made. Normally, at least 10 years' notice is given of any increase.
4 The Pensions Act 2014 requires governments to review the State Pension age (see reviews above). The March 2023 review confirmed the increase to age 67 but delayed making a decision on when the increase to 68 should be. The next review is due by 2025 (but may be delayed).

5 Pensioner spending includes expenditure on the state pension, pension credit, pensioner housing benefit and the winter fuel payment (now cut back).
6 Office for Budget Responsibility, *Welfare spending: pensioner benefits* (updated January 2024); *Economic and fiscal outlook – November 2023*. The figure for pensioner spending is forecast to increase to over £172 billion by the end of the decade. These figures are for Great Britain alone; Northern Ireland is assessed separately in *Northern Ireland social security*.
7 See gov.uk, Department of Work and Pensions, National statistics, *DWP benefits statistics: August 2023*. The August 2024 statistics have not updated the 2023 figures.
8 The Centre for Social Justice, chaired by Sir Iain Duncan Smith MP, in its report *Ageing Confidently* (2019).
9 The Labour Party manifesto for the 2019 General Election argued that the pension age should be fixed at 66 and any future increases abandoned. The June 2024 manifesto pledged to conduct a pensions review. This review was formally announced in July 2024, with the focus first on investment and then on improving pension outcomes and assessing retirement adequacy. Also in July 2024, the government announced a new Pension Schemes Bill. A petition to Parliament in 2024 argued for a State Pension age of 60.
10 See *JSNA Blackpool* (July 2022; August 2024).
11 Rest Less, *The number of over-seventies still working has more than doubled in a decade to nearly half a million in 2019* (May 2019, pre-pandemic), using the labour data from the Office for National Statistics.
12 See Trading Economics, *Retirement Age*; eportugal.gov.pt, *Who can request the old-age pension*.
13 See gov.uk, *State Pension*.
14 See gov.uk, *State Pension top up* (updated April 2014).
15 See gov.uk, Department for Work and Pensions, National statistics, *DWP benefits statistics: August 2023*. See Note 7.
16 See unbiased.co.uk, *Pension triple lock: what it is and why it is changing?*
17 See gov.uk, Policy paper, *State Pension age review 2023* (March 2023).
18 See gov.uk, *The basic State Pension*. Currently, the State Pension is increased annually by a Pensions Increase (Review) Order, enabled by the Social Security Pensions Act 1975.
19 See gov.uk, *Tax when you get a pension*.
20 In August 2024, Labour's Chancellor Rachel Reeves ruled out introducing (in the short term) national insurance on working pensioners' pay. The exemption for pensioners is designed, it is said, to encourage staying in work.
21 For full details, see House of Commons Library, *Health and Social Care Levy* (October 2022).
22 See Note 21.
23 See Health and Social Care Levy (Repeal) Act 2022.
24 See Note 6.
25 See ageuk.org.uk, *Pension Credit*.
26 See MoneySavingExpert, *Martin Lewis on pension credit: What over-66s need to know* (updated September 2024). However, when the winter fuel payment was abolished in July 2024, applications for Pension Credit rose sharply.
27 See gov.uk, *Pension Credit*.
28 See gov.uk, *DWP benefits statistics: August 2024* (August 2024). In Scotland, Attendance Allowance is being replaced by Pension Age Disability Payment.

29 See gov.uk, *Bereavement Support Payment*; see also Age UK, *Bereavement Support Payment*.
30 At 2024–25 rate.
31 See gov.uk, *Winter Fuel Payment* – amounts for 2023–24.
32 See tvlicensing.co.uk, *Over 75? Check if you can get a free TV Licence*.
33 See tvlicensing.co.uk, *Blind (severely sight impaired)*.
34 The Labour government has promised to introduce a Pensions Schemes Bill which will, amongst other things, introduce automatic consolidation of small pension pots (July 2024).
35 The Money Advice Service (now the MoneyHelper), *Pensions Dashboard Research* (May 2017).
36 Look carefully before you decide. See advice websites, such as Holly Boring Money and her article *How much has everyone else got in a pension?* (October 2023). But do your own research too.
37 See gov.uk, *Tax on your private pension contributions*.
38 For 2024–25, see The House of Commons Library, *Pension tax relief: The annual allowance and lifetime allowance* (April 2024).
39 See Note 34.
40 The Pension Schemes Act 2015, together with the Taxation of Pensions Act 2014. The minimum age of 55 is due to increase to 57 in 2028.
41 See gov.uk, *Private pension statistics commentary: July 2024* (July 2024).
42 UK Parliament, *Pension Scams* (March 2023), with a loss of £31 million from pension scams from 2017 to mid-2020.
43 Regulated before 2013 by the Financial Services Authority (FSA); from 2013, by the Prudential Regulatory Authority (PRA) and the Financial Conduct Authority (FCA). Check the Financial Services Register for regulated companies and individuals.
44 For an explanation of pensions dashboards and how they would work, see House of Commons Library, *Pensions dashboards* (August 2023).
45 Pension Dashboards, *Government response to the consultation* (Department for Work and Pensions, April 2019).
46 See gov.uk, *Government response: Draft Pensions Dashboards Regulations 2022* (July 2022).
47 The Pension Regulator, *Pensions dashboards: initial guidance* (updated April 2024).
48 See pensiondashboardsprogramme.org.uk, *Progress update report* (October 2023, updated April 2024); gov.uk, Department for Work and Pensions, Guidance, *Pensions dashboards: guidance on connection: the staged timetable* (March 2024).

CHAPTER 4
Inheritance Tax

1 For the current rules, see generally gov.uk, *How Inheritance Tax works: thresholds, rules and allowances*; boringmoney.co.uk, *Inheritance Tax for beginners: Everything you need to know* (October 2023).
2 See Office for Budget Responsibility, *Inheritance Tax* (April 2023; March 2024). The Institute for Fiscal Studies (IFS) forecasts that IHT revenue will increase to over £15 billion (in today's money and at today's thresholds) by

2032-33: *Reforming inheritance tax: Green Budget 2023* – Chapter 7 (September 2023). See also, gov.uk, *Inheritance Tax liabilities statistics: commentary* (July 2024).
3. Frozen at £325,000 since 2009 and currently set to remain fixed until at least 2030 (as stated in the October 2024 budget).
4. The average house price in the UK in 2023–2024 was £292,000, £309,000 in England: Office for National Statistics (ONS), *Private rent and house prices, UK: November 2024* (November 2024).
5. See gov.uk, *Inheritance nil-rate band and residence nil-rate band thresholds from 6 April 2026 to 5 April 2028* (November 2022); gov.uk, *Work out and apply the residence nil-rate band for Inheritance Tax* (updated September 2019). Claim for residence nil-rate band on Form IHT435.
6. See Note 5.
7. See Note 1.
8. See gov.uk, *Inheritance Tax reduced rate calculator*.
9. See HMRC, *Guide to completing your Inheritance Tax account* (IHT400) (2022) Notes).
10. See gov.uk, *Pay your Inheritance Tax bill*.
11. See Note 9 and Note 10.
12. As a starting point, try the free service of unbiased.co.uk to help you find a regulated financial adviser to suit your needs.
13. For meaning of 'direct descendants', see gov.uk, *Work out and apply the residence nil-rate band for Inheritance Tax* (updated September 2019); gov.uk, *Inheritance Tax Manual*, IHTM46034 (updated October 2024); HMRC, *Schedule IHT435*, Note 3.
14. From 2026, certain qualifying business and agricultural exemptions will be reduced by 50% and will therefore be taxed at 20% on assets exceeding £1 million in value. See for example the Octopus Inheritance Tax Service and the Octopus AIM Inheritance Tax Service. I am not endorsing any particular product; there are many others. AIM, the Alternative Investment Market, a sub-market of the London Stock Exchange, is designed to secure capital for smaller (sometimes riskier) businesses. It is less regulated than the main market.
15. OTS, *Inheritance Tax Review: Simplifying the design of Inheritance Tax* (second report, July 2019).
16. 4.39% of all deaths in the year 2021–22, up 17% on the previous year: gov.uk, *Inheritance Tax liabilities statistics: commentary* (updated July 2024). IFS, *Inheritance tax explained*: 'Around 5% of all deaths attracted IHT in 2022-23.'
17. AIM, the Alternative Investment Market: see Note 14.
18. See the Government's letter of response to the consultation: gov.uk, *Chancellor responds to OTS reports on Inheritance Tax and Capital Gains Tax* (30 November 2021). See also Note 14 for the 2024 autumn budget modification to certain IHT exemptions from 2026.
19. yougov.co.uk, *Inheritance* (September 2023).
20. See Note 2.

CHAPTER 5
Scams

1. Some of these tips come from Cyber Aware, a campaign website promoted by the Government: see ncsc.gov.uk, *Top tips for staying secure online* (reviewed December 2021). See also getsafeonline.org.
2. Passwords should be kept safely. Some people use a password manager, a computer programme for encrypted storage and ready access (for a fee). Companies include Dashlane, KeePass, Keeper, LastPass, NordPass, Norton and RoboForm.
3. actionfraud.police.uk, *A–Z of fraud*.
4. See gov.uk, *Fraud Strategy: stopping scams and protecting the public (accessible)* (May 2023); National Audit Office (NAO), *Progress combatting fraud* (November 2022); National Crime Agency, *Fraud*; UK Parliament, Committees, *Fraud*.
5. BT, *Communication Choices, Dealing with unwanted calls on your BT line*. See also ofcom.org.uk, *How to protect yourself from nuisance calls and messages*; iPhone User Guide, *Block or avoid unwanted calls on iPhone*.
6. See gov.uk, *Ban on cold calling for consumer financial services and products* (August 2023). See also *Fraud strategy*, Note 4.
7. Over £725 million in 2022; down to £708 million in 2023: UK Finance, *Annual Fraud Reports 2023* and *2024*.
8. Introduced in 2016 (2018 in Scotland).
9. Cifas, *This is Fraudscape 2024*: ID fraud in 2023 amounted to 64% of all fraud reports to the National Fraud Database.
10. See ONS, *Internet banking, by age group, Great Britain, 2019* (November 2019); Age UK, *"You can't bank on it anymore"* (May 2023).
11. The fraudulent use of contactless payment cards has led to banks withholding contactless transactions from time to time, requiring cards to be used occasionally with the PIN number.
12. There are a number of anti-phishing websites, such as fraudwatch.com and millersmiles.co.uk.
13. Thanks to the genuine TV Licensing website.
14. 393 such cases in 2018–19. See also National Crime Agency (NCA), *Fraud* (2023): 'Fraud against individuals is typically targeted at elderly and other vulnerable people, for whom consequences can be devastating – psychologically as well as financially.' See the University of Plymouth, *New report finds scammers are repeatedly targeting older people* (November 2023): most of these scams are phone related (landline, mobile or text), making people, particularly those living alone, feel unsafe in their own home.
15. See Action Fraud, *Spot the signs of ticket fraud* (April 2024).
16. The £75,000 figure is from 2021: UK Parliament, *Pension Scams* (March 2023). Before then, PMI reported (in November 2020) the average to be £82,000. Pensions Expert, however, reported a rather different average figure of £16,500 for 2020–2022. See also fca.org.uk, *Scammers target over £2m in pension pots in the last five months* (July 2021); gov.uk, *Pensions cold calling banned* (January 2019).
17. See Note 6, at paragraph 1.10.
18. See fca.org.uk, *Binary options scams* (updated March 2023).
19. August 2019.

20 AJ Bell, a pensions firm (January 2019).
21 fca.org.uk, *Retirement income market data 2021/22* (October 2022); *Retirement income market data 2022/23* (April 2024).
22 See UK Finance, *Annual Fraud Report 2024* (May 2024): down 5% on 2023.
23 UK Finance, *Annual Fraud Report 2023* (May 2023).
24 Payment Systems Regulator (PSR), *APP fraud performance data* (for 2023).
25 See psr.org.uk, *Confirmation of Payee, Response to our call for views CP21/6* (October 2021).
26 The Contingent Reimbursement Model (CRM) Code: see gov.uk, *Government approach to authorised push payment scam reimbursement* (May 2022). See also psr.org.uk, *Authorised push payment (APP) scams, Consultation paper* (November 2021); *Authorised push payment (APP) scams: Requiring reimbursement* (September 2022).
27 Section 72 of the Financial Services and Markets Act 2023 required the Payment Systems Regulator (PSR) to prepare and publish a draft requirement for mandatory reimbursement. See PSR, *APP scams* (March 2024). For the mandatory scheme, see PSR, *Specific Requirement 1 (FPS APP scam reimbursement rules)* and *Specific Direction 20 (FPS APP scam reimbursement requirement)* (both July 2024). In its review of APP scams, the PSR identified 429 cases in 2023 of losses over the new limit of £85,000: see PSR, *Authorised push payment (APP) scams performance* (July 2024).
28 The PSR has indicated that gross negligence equates with a significant degree of carelessness. HSBC, for example, may refuse reimbursement if the customer has been 'extremely careless' (October 2024). For an interesting analysis of the (then proposed) mandatory system from the banks' point of view, see solicitors Simmons & Simmons at simmons-simmons.com, *Confirmation of mandatory reimbursement for APP fraud* (June 2023).
29 The Financial Conduct Authority has in the past defined a vulnerable customer as 'Someone who, due to their personal circumstances, is especially susceptible to harm – particularly when a firm is not acting with appropriate levels of care.': see FCA, *FG21/1 Guidance for firms on the fair treatment of vulnerable customers* (February 2021).
30 Financial Ombudsman Service (FOS), *Fraud and scam complaints hit highest ever level* (September 2024).
31 See the film, *The Good Liar* (2019), with Helen Mirren and Ian McKellen.
32 See City of London Police at cityoflondon.police.uk, *Romance fraudsters break hearts and bank balances with £92.8 million lost in the last year* (October 2023). As with many fraud figures, statistics vary. For example, statistics from the UK Finance *Annual Fraud Report 2024*, report £36.5 million as the total loss for 2023 in over 4,100 cases, with an average loss of £8,700 per person. See also, ukfinance.org.uk, *Romance scams on the up during lockdown* (October 2022); CrimeStoppers, *Tackling romance fraud*.
33 crimestoppers-uk.org, *Romance fraud*.
34 Social Market Foundation, smf.co.uk, *Fraud is now Britain's dominant crime, but policing has failed to keep up* (March 2022).
35 actionfraud.police.uk has an online reporting tool, or call 0300 123 2040.
36 ONS describes it as the public-facing national fraud and cybercrime reporting centre; although only 13% of frauds against individuals are said to be reported to Action Fraud: NCA, National Strategy Assessment 2024, *Fraud*. See also Action Fraud, *Action Fraud roll out* (February 2013).

37 See gov.uk, *Fraud Strategy: stopping scams and protecting the public (accessible)* (May 2023).
38 *Which? Exclusive: scam victims ignored by police fraud reporting system* (September 2019).
39 Justice Committee report, *Fraud and the Justice System* (October 2022).
40 Oxford Academic, *Hiding behind the Veil of Action Fraud* (May 2021).
41 See gov.uk, *Fraud Strategy: stopping scams and protecting the public (accessible)* (May 2023).
42 uk.trustpilot.com (accessed 2 October 2024).
43 See Note 41, *Fraud Strategy* at p.19.
44 National Crime Agency (NCA), *Fraud*; see Note 4.
45 Age UK, *Scams and Fraud (England)* (April 2024). And see Note 4. NCA, National Strategic Assessment 2024, *Fraud*, has slightly different figures.
46 Social Market Foundation, *One in five people have been a victim of fraud* [in the UK and 14 other countries] *in the last couple of years, international survey finds* (March 2024); see also Statista, *Proportion of adults who were victims of fraud in England and Wales from April 2016 to March 2017 by age* (July 2017).
47 ONS, *Crime in England and Wales: year ending March 2019* (January 2020).
48 ONS, *Crime in England and Wales: year ending June 2024* (October 2024). See also assets.publishing.service.gov.uk, *The Scale and Nature of Fraud: A Review of the Evidence* (Home Office). And see Note 36.
49 See Notes 36, 37 and 48. The government's *Fraud Strategy* (May 2023) promised an extra 'over 400' specialist fraud investigators as part of a new National Fraud Squad.
50 National Audit Office (NAO), *Progress combatting fraud (November 2022); NAO, Tackling fraud and corruption against government* (March 2023), including an estimated £7.3 billion relating to temporary Covid-19 schemes.
51 Cyber crime is crime involving computers or the internet. For legal definitions, see the Fraud Act 2006, Computer Misuse Act 1990
52 ONS, *Crime in England and Wales: year ending 2023* (April 2024): on the Crime Survey for England and Wales (CSEW) fraud was down 16% on the previous year (particularly advance fee fraud), although fraud recorded by the police was up 1% in the same year, and computer misuse offences were up 29% according to CSEW. In the following year there was 'no statistically significant change': ONS, *Crime in England and Wales: year ending June 2024* (October 2024).
53 See Note 4.
54 The Labour Party Manifesto for the 2024 general election campaign included a promise to introduce 'a new expanded fraud strategy to tackle the full range of threats, including online, public sector and serious fraud'. See also Cifas, *A New Day, A New Government, A New Fraud Strategy* (July 2024).

CHAPTER 6
Health

1. University College London (UCL), *Uncovering clues to a healthy retirement – and it's not all lifestyle* (June 2018); *The Lancet*, Professor Eric J Brunner et al., *Midlife contributors to socioeconomic difference in frailty during later life: a prospective cohort study* (July 2018).
2. The Caerphilly Cohort Study (1979–2014); *International Journal of Epidemiology*, David Fone et al., *Cohort profile: the Caerphilly health and social needs electronic cohort study (E-CATALyST)* (December 2013).
3. See NHS, *Physical activity guidelines for older adults*.
4. *British Journal of Sports Medicine*, Dr Barbara Jefferis (UCL) et al., *Objectively measured physical activity, sedentary behaviour and all-cause mortality in older men: does volume of activity matter more than pattern of accumulation?* (February 2018).
5. World Health Organisation (WHO), *Physical activity* (October 2022). See also UK Chief Medical Officers, *Physical activity guidelines* (updated March 2023).
6. *European Heart Journal*, Joanna Blodgett (UCL) et al., *Device-measured physical activity and cardiometabolic health: the Prospective Physical Activity, Sitting, and Sleep (ProPASS) consortium* (February 2024).
7. *Neurology, Clinical Practice*, Joyce Gomes-Osman et al., *Exercise for cognitive brain health in ageing* (May 2018).
8. *British Journal of Sports Medicine*, Dr Jamie O'Driscoll (Canterbury Christ Church University), *Exercise training and resting blood pressure: a large-scale pairwise and network meta-analysis of randomised controlled trials* (July 2023). For exercises see many free demonstrations online and the helpful article in the *Guardian, The isometric secret: 15 ways to get much fitter – without moving a muscle* (8 August 2023).
9. *British Journal of Sports Medicine*, Dr Barbara Jefferis (UCL) et al., *Objectively measured physical activity, sedentary behaviour and all-cause mortality in older men: does volume of activity matter more than pattern of accumulation?* (February 2018).
10. *Cancer*, John Hopkins University School of Medicine, Catherine Handy Marshall et al., *Relation of Isolated Low High-Density Lipoprotein Cholesterol to Mortality and Cardiorespiratory Fitness* (May 2019). For prostate cancer, see *British Journal of Sports Medicine*, Dr Kate Bolam et al., *Association between change in cardiorespiratory fitness and prostate cancer incidence and mortality in 57, 652 Swedish men* (January 2024).
11. *British Medical Journal*, Norwegian School of Sport Sciences, Oslo, Ulf Ekelund, *Dose-response associations between accelerometry measured physical activity and sedentary time and all cause mortality: systematic review and harmonised meta-analysis* (August 2019). See also the *Journal of the American Medical Association (JAMA)*, Professor David Raichlen (University of Southern California), *Sedentary Behavior and Incident Dementia Among Older Adults* (September 2023).
12. See Note 4, Dr Jefferis. See also *British Journal of Sports Medicine*, Justin Lang et al., *Cardiorespiratory fitness is a strong and consistent predictor of morbidity and mortality among adults: an overview of meta-analyses representing over 20.9 million observations from 199 unique cohort studies* (May 2024)

13 American Academy of Neurology, *People who walk just 35 minutes a day may have less severe strokes* (September 2018).
14 NHS, *Benefits of exercise*.
15 WHO, *Physical activity* (June 2024).
16 Seneca, *Letters to Lucilius*.
17 See *International Journal of Geriatric Psychiatry*, Dr Anne Corbett (University of Exeter) et al., *An online investigation of the relationship between the frequency of word puzzle use and cognitive function in a larger sample of older adults* (May 2019).
18 See National Institutes of Health (NIH), Professor Debra Umberson (University of Texas) et al., *Social Relationships and Health: A Flashpoint for Health Policy* (August 2011); Harvard Health Publishing, *Get back your social life to boost thinking, memory and health* (October 2023). See also Age UK, *Social connections and the brain* (September 2022).
19 Celia Dodd, in the excellent *Not Fade Away: How to Thrive in Retirement* (Green Tree, 2018).
20 BDA, the Association of UK Dietitians, *Dieticians across the UK urge the public to avoid the diet rush this January* (December 2022).
21 See *The Diet Myth* (Weidenfeld & Nicholson, 2016), by Tim Spector, Professor of Genetic Epidemiology at King's College London, Honorary Consultant at Guy's and St Thomas' Hospital, London. See also Tim Spector, *Food for Life: The New Science of Eating Well* (Jonathan Cape, 2022).
22 Ibid.
23 See, for example, Obesity Action Scotland, *Obesity and Older People* (May 2022).
24 Cancer Research UK, *How does obesity cause cancer?* (February 2023).
25 See, for example, NHS Inform, *Health benefits of eating well*; nidirect, *Healthy eating for older adults*.
26 *The Lancet Diabetes & Endocrinology*, N Eckel et al., *Transition from metabolic healthy to unhealthy phenotypes and association with cardiovascular disease across BMI categories in 90,257 women (the Nurses' Health Study: 30-year follow-up from a prospective cohort study* (May 2018). See also *The Lancet Diabetes & Endocrinology*, CJ Lavie et al., *Obesity is rarely healthy* (May 2018); *The Lancet Diabetes & Endocrinology*, M Kivimaki et al., *Body-mass index and risk of obesity-related complex multimorbidity: an observational multicohort study* (March 2022).
27 For obesity in older life, see *Journal of Cachexia, Sarcopenia and Muscle*, Mark Burton et al., *Adiposity is associated with widespread transcriptional changes and downregulation of longevity pathways in aged skeletal muscle* (May 2023). For speedy eating, see *BMJ Open*, Y Hurst and H Fukuda (Kyushu University, Japan), *Effects of Changes in eating speed on obesity in patients with diabetes: a secondary analysis of longitudinal health check-up data* (February 2018). See also *Harvard Health Publishing, Slow down – and try mindful eating* (September 2022).
28 See, for example, *Journal of the American College of Cardiology*, Andrew Freeman, *A Clinician's Guide for Trending Cardiovascular Nutrition Controversies: Part II* (July 2018); WHO, *Healthy diet* (April 2020); nidirect.gov.uk, *Healthy eating for older adults*; gov.wales, *Food & Nutrition in Care Homes for Older People*; Age UK, *Healthy eating*; British Nutrition Foundation, *Older People* (2024).

29 See ibid., Andrew Freeman; *JAMA Internal Medicine*, E Loftfield et al., *Association of Coffee Drinking with Mortality by Genetic Variation in Caffeine Metabolism* (July 2018); *European Journal of Preventive Cardiology*, Professor Peter Kistler (Baker Heart and Diabetes Institute, Melbourne) et al., *The impact of coffee subtypes on incident cardiovascular disease, arrhythmias, and mortality: long-term outcomes from the UK Biobank* (November 2022); *Journal of Hypertension*, M Marozzi et al., *Coffee consumption relates to a reduction of vascular and heart damage in well-controlled hypertensives* (June 2023).

30 See Note 21, Professor Tim Spector at KCL.

31 *Mayo Clinic Proceedings*, Mercedes Sotos Prieto (Harvard TH Chan School of Public Health), *Adherence to a Mediterranean lifestyle associated with lower risk of all-cause and cancer mortality* (August 2023). *Molecular Psychiatry*, Dr Camille Lasalle (University College London) et al., *Healthy dietary indices and risk of depressive outcomes: a systematic review and meta-analysis of observational studies* (September 2018). See also *Molecular Nutrition & Food Research*, Alba Tor-Roca et al., *A Mediterranean Diet-Based Metabolomic Score and Cognitive Decline in Older Adults: A Case-Control Analysis Nested within the Three-City Cohort Study* (October 2023): The Mediterranean Diet is associated with healthy brain ageing (study of over 65s).

32 Ibid., Dr C Lasalle.

33 *The Lancet*, Professor J Mann (University of Otago, New Zealand) et al., *Carbohydrate quality and human health: a series of systematic reviews and meta-analyses* (January 2019). See also Academy of Nutrition Sciences, Kevin Whelan, Professor of Dietetics at King' College London, *Nature of the evidence base and approaches to guide nutrition interventions for individuals* (February 2024).

34 Andrew Mente, McMaster University, Ontario, presenting findings to the congress of the European Society of Cardiology in Munich (August 2018).

35 Dr Michelle Braude, author of *The Food Effect Diet* (Piatkus, 2017).

36 Professor Jeremy Pearson, Associate Medical Director, British Heart Foundation, quoted in the *Independent*, citing the Ontario study at Note 34 (August 2018).

37 The Scientific Advisory Committee on Nutrition (SACN) which advises Public Health England (August 2019).

38 National Institutes of Health (NIH), National Institute on Aging, *Healthy Meal Planning: Tips for Older Adults*.

39 UCL's Institute of Epidemiology and Health Care and University of Calgary and Alberta Health Services, Canada (August 2019).

40 *The Angina Monologues: stories of surgery for broken hearts* (Scribe UK, May 2019) by Samer Nashef.

41 See, for example, NHS, *Salt in your diet*; Action on Salt, *Salt and the older population*.

42 *The Lancet Public Health*, M Schwarzinger et al., *Contribution of alcohol use disorders to the burden of dementia in France 2008–13: a nationwide retrospective cohort study* (February 2018).

43 *Nature*, Medical Research Council, J Garaycoechea et al., *Alcohol and endogenous aldehydes damage chromosomes and mutate stem cells* (January 2018).

44 ONS, *Alcohol-specific deaths in the UK: registered in 2022* (April 2024): 10,048 deaths in 2022, the highest number on record; 32.8% higher than 2019.

45 Linda Bault, January 2018.
46 BMJ Open, Dr Mark Ashworth (King's College London), *Alcohol use, socio-economic deprivation and ethnicity in older people* (August 2015).
47 *The Lancet*, Dr Angela Wood (Cambridge University) et al., *Risk thresholds for alcohol consumption: combined analysis of individual-participant data for 599,912 current drinkers in 83 prospective studies* (April 2018).
48 See, for example, *BMC Medicine*, Yalan Tian et al., *Alcohol consumption and all-cause and cause-specific mortality among US adults: prospective cohort study* (June 2023).
49 *BMC Medicine*, Dara O'Neill (University College London), *Association of longitudinal alcohol consumption trajectories with coronary heart disease: a meta-analysis of six cohort studies using individual participant data* (August 2018). See also research at Queen's University Belfast (Andrew Kunxmann) published in *PLOS Medicine* (June 2018).
50 *Gastroenterology*, Caroline Le Roy, Tim Spector (both Kings College London) et al., *Red Wine Consumption Associated with Increased Gut Microbiota a-Diversity in Three Independent Cohorts* (January 2020); *Neurology*, Thomas Holland (Rush University Medical Centre) et al., *Association of Dietary Intake of Flavonols With Changes in Global Cognition and Several Cognitive Abilities* (November 2022). Cf. Warning that any level of alcohol consumption can increase risk of cardiovascular disease, in *Policy Brief*, World Heart Federation, Professor Monika Arora (January 2022).
51 *Journal of Studies on Alcohol and Drugs*, Vol.85, No.4, Dr Tim Stockwell et al., *Why Do Some Cohort Studies Find Health Benefits From Low-Volume Alcohol Use? A Systematic Review and Meta-Analysis of Study Characteristics That May Bias Mortality Risk Estimates* (July 2024). See also, NHS, *Drink less*; WHO (Europe), *No level of alcohol consumption is safe for our health* (January 2023).
52 *Apophthegms New and Old, as Originally Published in 1625*, Cambridge University Press (2013).
53 WHO, *Tobacco* (July 2023). See also White Paper, *Smoking Kills* (Cmnd.4177, December 1998).
54 Cancer Research UK, *Tobacco kills one person every five minutes* (May 2023).
55 Office for National Statistics (ONS), *Adult smoking habits in the UK: 2023* (October 2024); ONS, *Adult smoking habits in the UK: average cigarette consumption methodology* (June 2024).
56 *Addiction*, German D Carrasquilla (University of Copenhagen), et al., *Estimating causality between smoking and abdominal obesity by Mendelian randomization* (June 2024).
57 *European Heart Journal*, Lu Qi (Tulane University) et al., *Sleep patterns, genetic susceptibility, and incident cardiovascular disease: a prospective study of 385,292 UK biobank participants* (March 2020). See also *New Scientist*, Professor Kurt Lushington et al., *Multidimensional Sleep and Cardiometabolic Risk Factors for Type 2 Diabetes: Examining Self-Report and Objective Dimensions of Sleep* (November 2022); *Science Daily*, *Researchers identify distinct sleep types and their impact on long-term health* (March 2024).
58 *European Journal of Clinical Nutrition*, Haya Al Khatib (King's College London) et al., *The effects of partial sleep deprivation on energy balance: a systematic review and meta-analysis* (May 2017). See Sleep Foundation, *Nutrition and Sleep: Diet's Effect on Sleep* (updated May 2024).

59 See *Why We Sleep* (Penguin, 2017), by Matthew Walker, Professor of Neuroscience and Psychology at the University of California, Berkeley.

60 *Sleep Health*, Dr Victoria Garfield (MRC Unit for Lifelong Health & Ageing at UCL) et al., *Is there an association between daytime napping, cognitive function, and brain volume? A Mendelian randomization study in the UK Biobank* (October 2023). See also Mayo Clinic Proceedings and Mediterranean lifestyle at Note 31. For the view that people who take naps should see a GP, see *Alzheimer's & Dementia*, Yue Leng (University of California San Francisco) et al., *Daytime napping and Alzheimer's dementia: A potential bidirectional relationship* (January 2023).

61 *BMJ Open*, Daniel Kripke (Emeritus Professor of Psychiatry, University of California, San Diego) et al., *Hypnotics' association with mortality and cancer: a matched cohort study* (2012).

62 Sleep, Asher Rosinger (Penn State University, Pennsylvania) et ors, *Short sleep duration is associated with inadequate hydration: cross-cultural evidence from US and Chinese adults* (February 2019).

63 *Neurology and Urodynamics*, Junwei Wang (Wenzhou Medical University) et al., *Association between TV and/or video time and nocturia in adults: An analysis of the National Health and Nutrition Examination Survey* (February 2024).

64 Although a review of studies in 2024 found that claims that blue light disrupted sleep was overrated: *Sleep Medicine Reviews*, Michael Gradisar et al., *A bidirectional model of sleep and technology use: A theoretical review of How much, for whom, and which mechanisms* (August 2024).

65 See *European Journal of Clinical Nutrition*, Haya Al Khatib (King's College London) et al., *The effects of partial sleep deprivation on energy balance: a systematic review and meta-analysis* (May 2017). See Sleep Foundation, *Nutrition and Sleep: Diet's Effect on Sleep* (updated May 2024).

66 *Journal of Experimental Psychology: General*, Professor Michael Scullin et al., *The Effects of Bedtime Writing on Difficulty Falling Asleep: A Polysomnographic Study Comparing To-Do-Lists and Completed Activity Lists* (January 2018).

67 See Note 59, *Why We Sleep*. On 'binge sleeping', research presented to the European Society of Cardiology Congress in August 2024 (Yanjun Song, et al., Beijing, China) suggests that lie-ins at the weekend, after a troubled busy schedule reducing sleep during the week, may lower the risk of heart disease by one fifth.

68 See Note 59, *Why We Sleep*: Walker's suggestion at 18–18.5C.

69 See ONS, *Measuring National Well-being: At what age is Personal Well-being the highest?* (February 2016); ONS, *Measuring National Wellbeing: Quality of Life in the UK, 2018* (April 2018); ONS, *Personal and economic wellbeing in Great Britain: May 2021* (May 2021). See also Professor Richard Layard (London School of Economics) et al., *The Origins of Happiness: The Science of Wellbeing Over the Life Course* (Princeton University Press, 2018). See also, concerning social activity, *Psychology Ageing*, Denis Gerstorf (Humboldt University) et al., *Terminal Decline in Wellbeing: The Role of Social Orientation* (2016).

70 *Frontiers in Psychology*, Mary Carol Hunter (University of Michigan) et al., *Urban Nature Experiences Reduce Stress in the Context of Daily Life based on Salivary Biomarkers* (April 2019).

71 *BioScience*, Dr Andrea Mechelli (King's College London) et al., *Urban Mind: Using Smartphone Technologies to Investigate the Impact of Nature on Mental Wellbeing in Real Time* (February 2018).

72 Research by Saman Samadi (University of Victoria, Australia) et al., *Spontaneous generation of exogenous hydrogen peroxide by plants* (March 2023).
73 See, for example, *The Little Book of Hygge: The Danish Way to Live Well* by Meik Wiking (Penguin Books, 2016).
74 *European Journal of Cancer*, Samuel Smith (University of Leeds) et al., *Prevalence of beliefs about actual and mythical causes of cancer and their association with socio-demographic and health-related characteristics: Findings from a cross-sectional survey in England* (April 2018).
75 See NHS, *What is dementia*; UK Parliament, House of Lords library, *Dementia care* (January 2024). Alzheimer's Society has a higher figure of 982,000: see *Local Dementia Statistics*.
76 ONS, *Deaths registered in England and Wales: 2023* (October 2024).
77 WHO, *The top 10 causes of death* (August 2024) – the latest figures are for 2021.
78 *Nature Communications*, Professor Gwenaelle Douaud (Oxford University), et al., *The effects of genetic and modifiable risk factors on brain regions vulnerable to ageing and disease* (March 2024). On alcohol, compare one study in *Addiction*, Louise Mewton et al., *The relationship between alcohol use and dementia in adults aged more than 60 years: a combined analysis of prospective, individual-participant data from 15 international studies* (August 2022): abstinence from alcohol is associated with an increased risk for all-cause dementia; there is no consistent evidence amongst current drinkers that the amount of alcohol consumed in later life is associated with dementia risk. On pollution, see Report by the Committee on the Medical Effects of Air Pollutants (COMEAP), *Cognitive decline, dementia and air pollution* (July 2022); Air Quality Life Index (AQLI) 2024, *Annual Update* (August 2024).
79 *The Lancet Diabetes & Endocrinology*, Dr Nawab Qilbash (London School of Hygiene & Tropical Medicine) et al., *Does midlife obesity really lower dementia risk? – Authors' reply* (April 2015).
80 As reported in *The Times*, 22 August 2019.
81 See Alzheimer's Society, *How many people have dementia in the UK* (December 2021). See also WHO, *Dementia* (March 2023).
82 NHS, *Alzheimer's disease*.
83 NHS, *What is dementia*
84 *Brain*, Dennis Chan (University of Cambridge) et al., *Differentiation of mild cognitive impairment using an entorhinal cortex-based test of VR navigation* (May 2019). See also *Current Biology*, Professor Neil Burgess (UCL Institute of Cognitive Neuroscience) et al., *Overestimation in angular path integration precedes Alzheimer's dementia* (October 2023). For Tau PET brain imaging, see *Science Translational Medicine*, Gil Rabinovici et al., *Prospective longitudinal atrophy in Alzheimer's disease correlates with the intensity and topography of baseline tau-PET* (January 2020).
85 *Journal of American Geriatric Society*, Dr Justin Golub (Irving Medical Centre, Columbia University, New York), et al., *Observed Hearing Loss and Incident Dementia in a Multiethnic Cohort* (March 2017); Otol Nerotol, Justin Golub et al., *Hearing Loss and Incident Dementia: Claims Data From the New York SPARCS Database* (January 2022); *PLOS ONE*, Dr Piers Dawes (University of Manchester), et al., *Hearing Loss and Cognition: The Role of Hearing Aids, Social Isolation and Depression* (March 2015).

86 See gov.uk, Press release, *Lecanemab licensed for adult patients in the early stages of Alzheimer's disease* (August 2024); Alzheimer's Association, *Lecanemab Approved for Treatment of Early Alzheimer's Disease* (August 2024). Lecanemab was licensed by the Medicines & Healthcare products Regulatory Agency (MHRA) but refused prescription on the NHS by the National Institute for Health and Care Excellence (NICE). In July 2024 the European Medicines Agency (EMA) refused to licence lecanemab on the grounds that the benefits were both too small and were counterbalanced by possible serious side-effects. And for donanemab, see NICE, *New Alzheimer's treatment donanemab does not currently demonstrate value for the NHS says NICE* (October 2024).

87 *Nature Medicine*, Maxime Taquet (University of Oxford) et al., *The recumbent shingles vaccine is associated with lower risk of dementia* (July 2024).

88 *BMJ*, George Savva et al., *Anticholinergic drugs and risk of dementia: case-control study* (April 2018).

89 *PLOS Medicine*, Professor Clive Ballard (University of Exeter Medical School), with King's College London and Oxford Health NHS Foundation Trust, *Impact of person-centred care training and person-centred activities on quality of life, agitation, and antipsychotic use in people with dementia living in nursing homes: A cluster-randomised controlled trial* (February 2018).

90 See ibid., *PLOS Medicine*.

91 Such as Alzheimer's UK, Dementia Friends, Dementia UK, Dementia Carers, Contented Dementia Trust.

92 The late Wendy Mitchell, author of *Somebody I used to know* (Bloomsbury, 2018).

93 Dr Sara Imarisio (November 2019); see also Alzheimer's Research UK, *Heart conditions linked with an increased risk of dementia*: 'What's good for your heart is also good for your head.' (Dr Imarisio, June 2022).

94 *Alzheimer's & Dementia: The Journal of the Alzheimer's Association*, Dr Adam Boxer et al., *Active lifestyles moderate clinical outcomes in autosomal dominant frontotemporal degeneration* (January 2020). For reading, see The Reading Agency, *Reading Well for dementia*.

95 WHO, *Dementia* (March 2023).

96 *BLJ*, Hong Chen (Oxford University) et al., *Dementia and Physical Activity (DAPA) trial of moderate to high intensity exercise training for people with dementia: randomised controlled trial*: High intensity exercise, as opposed to moderate exercise, may actually increase mental decline (May 2018).

97 *JAMA*, Cecilia Samieri et al., *Association of Cardiovascular Health Level in Older Age with Cognitive Decline and Incident Dementia* (August 2018).

98 *New England Journal of Medicine*, Dr John McNeil (Monash University, Melbourne) et al., *Effect of Aspirin on Disability-free Survival in the Healthy Elderly* (September 2018).

99 *Neurology*, Miguel Arce Renteria (Columbia University Medical Centre), et al., *Illiteracy, dementia risk, and cognitive trajectories among older adults with low education* (November 2019). *International Journal of Geriatric Psychiatry*, Anne Corbett, Professor of Dementia Research (University of Exeter), et al., *The relationship between playing musical instruments and cognitive trajectories: Analysis from a UK ageing cohort* (January 2024).

100 *Nature Ageing*, Dr Andrew Sommerlad (UCL Psychiatry), *Social participation and risk of developing dementia* (May 2023). See also *British Journal of Psychiatry*, Andrew Steptoe (University College London), et al., *Cultural en-*

gagement and cognitive reserve: museum attendance and dementia incidence over a ten-year period (November 2018); Professor Richard Restak, author of *How to Prevent Dementia* (Penguin Life 2023); *BMC Medicine*, Dr Hamish Foster et al., *Social connection and mortality in UK Biobank: a prospective cohort analysis* (November 2023); *Communications Psychology*, Gillian Sandstrom and Lara Aknin, *People are surprisingly reluctant to reach out to old friends* (April 2024).

101 *Nature Human Behaviour, Positive association between Internet use and mental health among adults aged >50 years in 23 countries*, Professor Qingpeng Zhang, The University of Hong Kong, et al. (November 2024).

CHAPTER 7
Home

1 Office for National Statistics (ONS), *Families and households in the UK: 2023* (May 2024), an 8% increase on 2022. See also ONS, *Profile of the older population living in England and Wales and changes since 2011* (April 2023).
2 See NHS, *Carbon monoxide poisoning*; and the National Institute for Health and Excellence (NICE), *Carbon monoxide poisoning* (revised June 2023).
3 The London Fire Brigade (LFB), for example, will make a home fire-safety visit and fit free smoke alarms there and then, if you need them. So too will the West Midlands Fire Service. They provide Safe and Well visits (previously known as home safety checks).
4 These are all commercial products. For helpful details and recommended products see Age Space, *Assistive Technology for the Elderly: A Guide to Getting Started*; Independent Age, *Getting help at home*; Age UK: Digital fall alarm.
5 See NHS (www.nhs.uk), *Getting a care needs assessment*; and gov.uk, *Apply for a needs assessment by social services*.
6 See, for example, rica.org.uk, *Features & Reviews*. RICA, the Research Institute for Disabled Consumers, is a UK charity providing independent research on accessible products and services. It describes easy-to-use appliances, such as for bathing, accessible heating controls and energy saving options, with the purpose of making life at home much simpler.
7 See gov.uk, *Disabled Facilities Grants*; gov.scot, *Independent Living, Equipment and adaptations*.
8 See also the Edward Gostling Foundation.
9 See, for example, Independent Age, Living Made Easy and MoneyHelper.
10 See Independent Age, *Getting help at home*.
11 See also the Royal Horticultural Society at rhs.org.uk.
12 *The Gentle Art of Swedish Death Cleaning: How to Free Yourself and Your Family from a Lifetime of Clutter*, by Margareta Magnusson (Simon & Schuster, 2018).
13 For example, the homelessness charity St Mungo's, will accept a range of goods, in addition to clean clothing. You can donate to any of Oxfam's 550 high street shops or by post. The Salvation Army has 8,000 clothing banks in the UK. See also, for example, Age UK, Sue Ryder, Scope, British Red Cross, RSPCA, and many hospice charities.
14 For example, West Sussex Council accept second-hand books at all 12 of their recycling centres.

15 *A Monk's Guide to a Clean House and Mind* (Penguin, 2018).
16 See Good Housekeeping, *Ten Best Indoor Plants for Your Health, According to Research* (July 2022).
17 Leeds Homeshare, for example, is a Leeds City Council scheme that matches 'a householder, who has a spare room and needs a bit of support with daily tasks and chores', with 'a home sharer, who can give them ten hours of support per week in exchange for accommodation at a low cost'.
18 In London, for example, the Helpful Housemates scheme does something similar, matching the householder with a lodger. Their team vets for suitable candidates and can help out if issues arise. Helpful Housemates, one of many such organisations, is part of Share and Care Homeshare, a Community Interest Company (CIC). Homeshare UK is a UK network for some 20 Homeshare organisations in different parts of the country.
19 See gov.uk, *Rent a room in your home*.
20 Legal advice on the content of an agreement might be a good idea.
21 See gov.uk, *Shared ownership homes: buying improving and selling*; HM Government, *Own Your Home, Older Persons Shared Ownership (OPSO)*. There are different rules on shared ownership in Wales, Northern Ireland and Scotland.
22 See the NHS website, www.nhs.uk, *Moving to a new home: housing options for older people or people with disabilities*. If you are looking for sheltered housing, the links in this website will direct you to the website of your local council. Very sheltered housing or extra care housing, unlike most sheltered housing, is regulated by the Care Quality Commission. See also the UK Cohousing Network at cohousing.org.uk.
23 In *Specialist housing for older people*, Age UK provides links to the charities Abbeyfield which has a number of retirement living options and the Almshouse Association which provides self-sufficient, low-cost community housing.
24 The charity Elderly Accommodation Counsel (EAC) provides a free helpline to give you an informed choice about your housing or care needs. They also offer directories of accommodation and services throughout the UK.

CHAPTER 8
Care

1 The Nuffield Trust (an independent health think tank), *The decline of publicly funded social care for older adults* (March 2023).
2 CQC, *The state of health care and adult social care in England 2023/24* (October 2024): as at March 2024.
3 The National Audit Office, nao.org.uk, *The adult social care market in England* (March 2021).
4 See Note 1.
5 homecare.co.uk, *Home care statistics: number of providers, service users & workforce* (updated June 2024).
6 statista.com, *Number of people living in care homes in the United Kingdom in 2022, by country* (November 2023). ONS, *Older people living in care homes in 2021 and changes since 2011* (October 2023): 278,946 people aged 65 and over living in care homes in England and Wales in 2021 (82.1% of all care home residents in England and Wales).

7 The National Audit Office, nao.org.uk, *The adult social care market in England* (March 2021). See also ONS, *Unpaid care by age, sex and deprivation, England and Wales: Census 2021* (February 2023). According to ONS, in 2021 there were approximately 128,200 unpaid carers aged between 5 and 17 years in England and Wales. One report suggests that nearly 25% of those aged 65 or over in 2016–17 received 'some sort of informal care'. In addition, it has been estimated that one in three NHS staff in England are also unpaid carers: Carers UK (April 2021).
8 See Note 3.
9 Research by Carers UK.
10 See nhs.co.uk, *Help at home from a paid carer*.
11 See NHS, *Getting a care needs assessment*; gov.uk, *Apply for a needs assessment by social services*.
12 Nuffield Trust, Note 1: in the year 2021–22, 33% of adults had to wait more than six months for an assessment. See Independent Age, *Care needs assessments*.
13 According to homecare.co.uk, there are over 10,000 home care providers in the UK, all regulated.
14 See nhs.co.uk, *Help at home from a paid carer*. This provides a link to homecare services and agencies in your area, as well as a long alphabetical list of national homecare providers in England, with information on each and their services. A local search may not bring up a national provider. The CQC can help too: see cqc.org.uk, *Find homecare agencies* and *Find and compare services*.
15 cqc.org.uk, *Our ratings and scores* (updated September 2024); see also CQC, *Ratings: adult social care services* (updated May 2022). All individuals and organisations providing health or adult social care activities in England must register with the CQC: see the Health and Social Care Act 2008 and the Health and Social Care Act 2008 (Regulated Activities) Regulations 2014.
16 homecare.co.uk claims to review over 13,000 homecare and residential care providers: see *Reviews for Home Care, Live in Care & Nursing Care Providers*. You can search by location or provider name.
17 See cqc.org.uk, *Scope of registration* (updated February 2024); and the Health and Social Care Act 2008 (Regulated Activities) Regulations 2014.
18 See also gov.uk, *Employ someone: step by step*.
19 See gov.wales, *Charging for social care*.
20 See homecare.co.uk, *Paying for home care in Northern Ireland in 2024* (updated May 2024).
21 For helpful details, see agescotland.org.uk, *Care and Support at Home: Assessment and Funding*; Independent Age, *Care needs assessments*. See the Community Care and Health (Scotland) Act 2002.
22 See gov.uk, *Carer's Allowance: How it works*.
23 In April 2024 a financial inclusion commissioner resigned from the Prime Minister's Dementia Friendly Communities Champion Group because the burden rested on the carer to declare overclaiming (often accidental), despite the DWP being data rich. In October 2024, the Starmer government announced an independent review into 'overpayments' of Carer's Allowance.
24 See nhs.uk, *Carer's assessments* [sic]; *Carers' breaks and respite care*.
25 A number of charities, such as The Respite Association (respiteassociation.org), Carefree Space (carefreespace.org), Parkinson's UK (parkinsons.org.

uk) provide short breaks or respite funding for carers. For more detail see disability-grants.org.
26 Nuffield Trust, above: in December 2022, 18% of patients were delayed waiting for a care or nursing home bed. 25% were waiting for a home care package.
27 See Notes 5, 16 and 20.
28 The UK Care Guide, which describes itself as a 'comprehensive resource hub', suggests a lower range of £600 to £950: see *Paying for care home fees in the UK* (November 2024).
29 The King's Fund, *Social Care 360: Workforce and Carers* (March 2024); *Beyond Dilnot: the need for wider reform* (May 2013); homecare.co.uk, *Home care facts and stats: number of providers, service users & workforce* (June 2024): over 800,000 care workers in the UK, providing home care in the UK to more than 950,000 people.
30 CQC, *State of care 2022/23* (updated October 2024).
31 CQC, *The state of health and adult social care in England 2023/24, Appendix: CQC ratings charts* (October 2024). As at August 2024, 17% required improvement (up 5% on previous data) and 1% were inadequate. See also the National Audit Office, nao.org.uk, *The adult social care market in England (March 2021)*: figures relating to May 2020 (15% required improvement; 1% were inadequate).
32 The National Audit Office, nao.org.uk, *The adult social care market in England* (March 2021).
33 Age UK report (February 2020).
34 See Report by Institute for Fiscal Studies (IFS), *Adult social care in England: what next?* (October 2024). See also the National Audit Office (NAO), *Reforming adult social care in England* (November 2023).
35 See Health and Social Care (Reform) Act (Northern Ireland) 2009; Health and Social Care Act (Northern Ireland) 2022; Public Bodies (Joint Working) (Scotland) Act 2016; Social Services and Well-being (Wales) Act 2014 and Well-being of Future Generations (Wales) Act 2015.
36 See gov.uk, Guidance, *Social care – charging for care and support: local authority circular* (February 2024).
37 Note 1, The Nuffield Trust.
38 ONS, *Care homes and estimating the self-funding population, England: 2021 to 2022* (July 2023).
39 See Note 31 NAO.
40 See gov.uk, Competition and Markets Authority, *Care homes market study* (updated March 2018).
41 NAO, *Reforming adult social care in England* (November 2023).
42 *Fairer Care Funding*, the Dilnot Report of the Commission on Funding of Care and Support (July 2011). Some of the Dilnot recommendations were brought into force by the Care Act 2014.
43 See gov.uk, Policy paper, *Build Back Better: Our Plan for Health and Social care* (September 2021, updated September 2024)
44 Nuffield Trust, above. 1.37 million requests in 2021–22, up from 1.31 million in 2015–16.
45 See Note 42, Dilnot, *Fairer Care Funding*.
46 Compared with public spending on health, which increased by over 10% in the same period: see references at Note 34.

47 nao.org.uk, *The adult social care market in England* (March 2021).
48 See Notes 31 and 32, NAO.
49 nidirect.gov.uk, *Your home, assets and residential care or nursing home fees*.
50 See gov.wales, *Charging for social care*.
51 See the Social Services and Wellbeing (Wales) Act 2014; Alzheimer's Society, *Who pays for care home fees in Wales?*
52 For helpful details, see agescotland.org.uk, *Care and Support at Home: Assessment and Funding*; Independent Age, *Care needs assessments*; *Get a Care Needs Assessment*. See the Community Care and Health (Scotland) Act 2002.
53 Care Information Scotland, careinfoscotland.scot, *Paying care home fees* (June 2024).
54 See Note 42, Dilnot *Fairer care funding*.
55 Although some steps taken towards integration include the creation of Health and Wellbeing Boards (see Health and Social Security Act 2012); the establishment of the Better Care Fund; and the symbolic renaming of the Department of Health as the Department of Health and Social Care (2018).
56 See the Health and Care Act 2022 which provides the foundations for a more joined-up system at a local level.
57 See Note 29, The King's Fund.
58 Legislated by Parliament as the Health and Social Care Levy Act 2021.
59 See gov.uk press release, *Record £36 billion investment to reform NHS and Social Care* (7 September 2021).
60 White Paper, *Integration and innovation: working together to improve health and social care for all* (February 2021).
61 Secretary of State for Health and Social Care, statement to House of Commons (22 September 2022). A further £250 million was announced in January 2023. See also gov.uk, *Health and Social Care Secretary sets out plan for patients with new funding to bolster social care over winter* (September 2022).
62 Chancellor Hunt's Autumn Statement (November 2022); Chancellor Reeves' Statement, 29 July 2024. See also House of Commons Library, *Proposed adult social care charging reforms (including cap on care costs)* (November 2022); with provision for a cap already set out in the Care Act 2014 (as amended by the Health and Care Act 2022); and House of Commons Library, *Introducing a cap on care costs* (July 2024); House of Lords Library, *Social care in England: Current situation, case for a strategy and further support for unpaid carers* (September 2024). See also gov.uk, *Operational guidance to implement a lifetime cap on care costs* (updated January 2023).

CHAPTER 9
Rights

1 Gwyneth Jones, a 77-year-old Australian woman, who made claims against her retirement facility which she had lived in for more than a decade.
2 See ONS, *Living longer: Is the age of 70 the new age 65?* (November 2019): ONS refers to 65 as the 'traditional age as the marker for the start of older age'. See also NHS England, *Improving care for older people*.
3 Estimates for mid-2022: see ONS, *Population estimates for the UK, England, Wales, Scotland, and Northern Ireland: mid-2023* (October 2024). Detailed estimate for those aged 65 and over is 12,736,451.

4 ONS, Dataset: *Estimates of the population for the UK, England, Wales, Scotland, and Northern Ireland* (March 2024); 10,841,000 (mid-2012), 12,736,451 (mid-2022).
5 ONS, *Overview of UK population: August 2019* (August 2019). See also ONS, *Overview of the UK population: 2020* (February 2022).
6 There is also a UN Open-Ended Working Group, started in 2010 as a data collection and discussion forum. Its 14th Session was held in May 2024 and recommended the possible option of a UN Convention to protect the human rights of older persons. But talks on a convention have progressed slowly. There is also a UN Independent Expert on the Rights of Older Persons.
7 UN Department of Economic and Social Affairs, *World Social Report 2023: Leaving No One Behind in an Ageing World.*
8 UN, *Political Declaration and Madrid International Plan of Action on Ageing (MIPAA). See also the UN Brasilia Declaration (2007); the UN San Jose Charter on the Rights of Older Persons in Latin America and the Caribbean (2012).*
9 Charter of Fundamental Rights of the EU, Article 25.
10 See proposal in *European Charter of the rights and responsibilities of older people in need of long-term care and assistance* (June 2010).
11 Article 21.
12 Article 25.
13 See the European Union (Withdrawal) Act 2018.
14 The centrepiece of the Council of Europe is the European Convention on Human Rights (ECHR) and the European Court of Human Rights. The Council of Europe is a 46-member state body (the Russian Federation withdrew on 25 February 2022 when it invaded Ukraine and Belarus was suspended for supporting Russia). The United Kingdom is a member state and was one of the 10 founder members. By contrast, in terms of numbers, the EU has 27 member states. The ECHR plays a central role in the arrangements for power-sharing in Northern Ireland: see *The Belfast Agreement*, otherwise known as the Good Friday Agreement (1998).
15 Recommendation CM/Rec(2014)2.
16 The words 'such as ...' before the list indicate that the list is not closed. See European Court of Human Rights, *Guide on Article 14 of the European Convention of Human Rights and of Article 1 to Protocol No.12 to the Convention, Prohibition on discrimination* (updated August 2022): The European Court has recognised that age constitutes 'other status' for the purposes of Article 14, but has not, to date, suggested that discrimination on ground of age should be equated with other grounds of discrimination (para.151). See also EU Directive 2000/78/EC.
17 Private Member's Bill, *Commissioner for Older People (Scotland) Bill* (June 2023).
18 In England the post of Commissioner for Older People has been proposed and championed by campaigning charities such as Age UK, Independent Age and the Centre for Ageing Better.
19 See Commissioner for Older People for Northern Ireland (COPNI); the Commissioner for Older People (Northern Ireland) Act 2011; and the COPNI *Corporate Plan 2022–2024*.
20 See *Older People's Commissioner for Wales (Comisiynydd Pobl Hyn Cymru)*; Commissioner for Older People (Wales) Act 2006 and the Commissioner for Older People in Wales Regulations 2007.

21 See olderpeople.wales.
22 olderpeople.wales; copni.org.
23 See humanrights.gov.au, Australian Human Rights Commission, *Age Discrimination* (2024).
24 Health & Disability Commissioner, *Aged Care Commissioner* (2024); *Amplifying the voices of older people across Aotearoa New Zealand* (March 2024).
25 Department of Social Justice and Empowerment, Government of India, *Senior Citizen Division*.
26 See UN Economic and Social Commission for Asia and the Pacific: unescap.org, People's Republic of China, *Legislation and National Polices on Older Persons*.
27 See UK Parliament, Committees, *The rights of older people*. There is one House of Commons select committee (with at least 11 MPs) for each Government department, scrutinising spending, policies and administration. A select committee reports publicly to the House of Commons and usually requires a response from Government. See parliament.uk, *Select Committees*.
28 The All-Parliamentary Group (APPG) is supported by the charity Age UK. It ceased to exist after the dissolution of Parliament in 2024, but is expected to be reconstituted. An APPG is a cross-party forum and holds meetings to discuss relevant issues.
29 See *Ex parte Witham* [1998] QB 575. See Michael Fordham QC's excellent article *Common Law Rights, Judicial Review*, Vol. 16 (1) (2011).
30 See *Ex parte Doody* [1994] 1 AC 531.
31 See *R (Q) v. Secretary of State for the Home Department* [2003] EWCA Civ 364. The Universal Declaration of Human Rights was proclaimed by the UN General Assembly on 10 December 1948.
32 See Note 14, European Convention.
33 As amended by Part 2, Chapter 2, of the Mental Health Act 2007, particularly relating to Deprivation of Liberty safeguards.
34 See gov.uk, *Code of practice: Mental Health Act 1983* (updated October 2017). See also nhs.uk, *Mental Health Act*; gov.uk, *Reforming the Mental Health Act: summary* (August 2021), which makes proposals for legislative reform which include, amongst others, *giving patients more rights to challenge detention* and *making sure patients are viewed and treated as rounded individuals*.
35 See NHS England, *Feedback and complaints to NHS England*; nhsinform.scot, *Making a complaint about your NHS care or treatment*; gov.wales, *NHS Wales complaints and concerns: Putting Things Right*; nidirect.gov.uk, *How to complain or raise concerns about health services*.
36 *R (Adath Yisroel Burial Society) v HM SC for Inner North London* [2018] EWHC 969 (Admin) at [114].
37 Sections 4, 5, 149(7), Equality Act 2010.
38 Section 4, Equality Act 2010.
39 Introduced by the Employment (Age) Regulations 2006 (see the Equal Treatment Framework Directive 2000/78); now superseded by the Equality Act 2010.
40 Paragraph 19, explanatory notes to Equality Act 2010. Regulation 3, Employment Equality (Age) Regulations (Northern Ireland) 2006.
41 See acas.org.uk, *Age Discrimination: key points for the workplace* (February 2019).

42 Section 13, Equality Act 2010.
43 Section 19, Equality Act 2010.
44 Section 26, Equality Act 2010.
45 Section 27, Equality Act 2010.
46 This provision applies only to adults aged 18 and over: section 28(1)(a), Equality Act 2010. See gov.uk guidance from the Government Equalities Office including *Banning Age Discrimination in Services: An overview for service providers and customers* and *The Equality Act, making equality real* (an Easy Read Document).
47 Section 13(2), Equality Act 2010.
48 See the Supreme Court case of *Seldon v Clarkson Wright and Jakes (A Partnership)* [2012] UKSC 16, a case of direct discrimination.
49 *Ewart v University of Oxford*, 3324911/2017 (20 December 2019): the professor was 69. *N Field-Johnson et ors. v. University of Oxford*, 3301882/2020 (9 March 2023). Cf. *Pitcher v University of Oxford*, 3323858/2016 (16 May 2019) came to the contrary conclusion. Combined appeals in the cases of *Pitcher* and *Ewart* were dismissed by the Employment Appeal Tribunal: [2021] IRLR 946.
50 See the case of *Seldon* in Note 48.
51 Equality and Human Rights Commission, *Employment: Code of Practice* (September 2015).
52 Sections 149, 150 and Schedule 19, Equality Act 2010; the Equality Act 2010 (Specific Duties) Regulations 2011. See also gov.uk, *Public sector equality duty* (July 2012); *Public Sector Equality Duty: guidance for public authorities* (December 2023).
53 Baroness Hale of Richmond in *Ghaidan v Godin-Mendoza* [2004] UKHL 30; [2004] 2 AC 557, at para.132.
54 See Older People's Commissioner for Wales website: *Taking Action Against Ageism*.
55 See the Government good practice guidance, at gov.uk, Department for Culture, Media & Sport, *Asking and responding to questions of discrimination in the provision of goods and services and public functions* (January 2014). These questions and answers may resolve the complaint or help you in making one.
56 For 'injury to feelings', see Vento compensation bands (from April 2024).
57 Section 124(2)(c), Equality Act 2010.
58 Age UK's analysis of data from the 2019 British Election Study, *Post-Election Random Probability Survey*.
59 See House of Commons, *Voter ID*; the Voter Identification Regulations 2022.
60 See gov.uk, *Apply for photo ID to vote (called a 'Voter Authority Certificate')*. This applies in England, Wales and Scotland. Northern Ireland has had the photo ID requirement since 2003: see The Electoral Office for Northern Ireland (EONI), *Electoral Identity Card FAQs*.
61 Section 2, Suicide Act 1961. For Bill procedure, see Hansard Society, *The Assisted Dying Bill: A guide to the Private Member's Bill process* (November 2024). A similar Bill, the Assisted Dying for Terminally Ill Adults (Scotland) Bill was introduced in Scotland in 2024.

CHAPTER 10
After Death

1. *Financial Times* (5 May 2018).
2. A modern haiku (Isobar Press, 2022).
3. Births and Deaths Registration Act 1953.
4. For meaning of natural causes see *R (Touche) v Inner London North Coroner* [2001] 1 QB 1206: death is unnatural when it is not natural; often unnatural means little more than abnormal or unexpected.
5. The number of deaths in England and Wales has risen from 530,000 in 2019 to about 580,000 deaths in 2023: see *Coroner Statistics 2023* (May 2024).
6. See mygov.scot, *Register a death* (2019).
7. See moneyhelper.org.uk, *Help paying for a funeral*. See also Competition and Markets Authority (CMA) investigation into funeral prices (updated July 2021) at gov.uk, *Funerals Market Study*; and *Welcome to the SunLife Cost of Dying Report 2024*: SunLife, the life insurance company, estimates 'the cost of dying' (funeral expenses, professional fees and other costs) at over £9,500 (as at 2023). By comparison, co-oplegalservices.co.uk assessed the average cost in 2019 as just under £4,000: see *Can You Pay Funeral Expenses Out of the Estate* (March 2020).
8. At quakersocialaction.org.uk.
9. See gov.uk, *Get help with funeral costs (Funeral Expenses Payment)*; gov.uk, *Benefits and financial support when someone dies*.
10. There are few laws of general application to burial grounds. Most burial law is directed at particular types of burial grounds, such as those operated by local authorities (the Local Authorities' Cemeteries Order 1977 (LACO), as amended) or the Church of England (various ecclesiastical measures, although the law relating to churchyards is mostly common law). Individual burial grounds may also be subject to private Acts of Parliament. See assets.publishing.service.uk, *Guide for Burial Ground managers* (Department for Constitutional Affairs, November 2005); assets.publishing.service.uk, *Natural burial grounds, Guidance for operators* (Ministry of Justice, 2009).
11. See gardens-of-peace.org.uk.
12. See Environment Agency (EA), *Funeral practices, spreading ashes and caring for the environment*. Contact the EA on 0870 850 6506 or by email at inquiries@environment-agency.gov.uk. See also the helpful guidance from The National Death Centre, *Independent Funeral Advice, Private land burial* (April 2010).
13. Quoted in *The Funniest Thing You Never Said* (Ebury Press, 2004).
14. See Cremation (England and Wales) Regulations 2008, amended by Cremation (England and Wales) (Amendment) Regulations 2016 and 2017. See also Institute of Cemetery and Crematorium Management (ICCM) at iccm-uk.com.
15. The Cremation Society, cremation.org.uk, *Progress of Cremation in the British Islands*, 1885–2023.
16. Updated September 2024. These forms (and others) originate from the Cremation (England and Wales) Regulations 2008, as amended, from March 2022, by the Cremation (England and Wales) (Amendment) Regulations 2022. See also the Cremation Act 1902.
17. See gov.scot, *Cremation: statutory forms* (updated January 2023).

18 City of Belfast Crematorium; Antrim and Newtownabbey Crematorium.
19 See Environment Agency, *Funeral practices, spreading ashes and caring for the environment*, above.
20 See gov.uk, *Applying for probate*.
21 For guidance on using a probate practitioner, see moneyhelper.org.uk, *When to use a professional firm for probate and estate administration*.
22 See the Notification of Deaths Regulations 2019, as amended by the Cremation, Coroners and Notification of Deaths (England and Wales) Regulations 2024 and the Medical Certificate of Cause of Death Regulations 2024.
23 See the Medical Examiners (England) Regulations 2024 and the Medical Examiners (Wales) Regulations 2024. For coroner statistics, see gov.uk, *Coroners Statistics 2023: England and Wales* (May 2024).

Appendix

1 There are plenty of free templates online. See, for example, mydecisions.org.uk, now the charity Compassion in Dying, *Advance Decision Pack* and *Advance Statement*; gov.uk, *Model Advance Decision, Form F*; Alzheimer's Society at alzheimers.org.uk, *Download a free template of an advance decision form* and *Advance statement and dementia*; Bereavement Advice Centre, *Download a sample advance decision & statement document*. See also nhs.co.uk, *Advance decision to refuse treatment (living will)* and *Advance statement about your care wishes*. The Annex is in part with thanks to mydecisions.org.uk (now Compassion in Dying).
2 Section 4(6), Mental Capacity Act 2005, requires the person's 'past and present wishes and feelings' to be taken into account.
3 See also Organ Donation Scotland and Organ Donation Northern Ireland for registration as a donor in those countries.

Acknowledgements

My particular thanks go to my superb agent, Jüri Gabriel. He secured a great home for this book at the splendid Bedford Square Publishers. The excellent Carolyn Mays, leading the team, has skilfully guided me through to publication.

Thanks, too, for Sophie Lazar's constructive and detailed editing, Nicky Barneby's lucid design and typeset, and Polly Halsey at BSP for innovative production.

My wife, Suzie Dalal, has been as ever a guiding light, inspiration and critically discerning editor at the writing stage. Thanks to our son Dan Thornton for looking at some of the modern tech stuff and to our daughter Amy Thornton on health.

I am also hugely grateful to a galaxy of experienced and well-informed experts who have encouraged me and put me right on a range of difficult topics: Alex Ruck Keene KC (Hon), Visiting Professor King's College London; Geraldine Van Bueren KC, Professor Emerita Queen Mary University of London, Hon Senior Fellow British Institute of International and Comparative Law and Visiting Fellow Kellogg College Oxford; Karon Monaghan KC; Philippa Barton, Director Duncan Lewis Solicitors; Daniel Wackett, Independent Financial Adviser, Managing Director Altorfer Financial Management Limited; David Sutton, Head of Wealth Planning Support Brown Shipley; Simon Mitchell, Partner and Head of Wills, Estates and Tax Planning Thomson, Snell & Passmore LLP.

About the Author

His Honour Sir Peter Thornton KC was a practising barrister in human rights law, a QC (now KC), founder member and head of Doughty Street Chambers, a Senior Circuit Judge at the Old Bailey (the Central Criminal Court) and the first Chief Coroner of England and Wales.

He is now a Visiting Professor at King's College London, a member of the Independent Expert Panel of the House of Commons, chair of the University College London Discipline Review Body, and international trainer of coroners with the Civil Service College and the Commonwealth Magistrates and Judges Association. He has written and edited numerous published works, and broadcast regularly on civil liberty issues and criminal law and coroner law on programmes such as *Newsnight*, *The Today Programme* on Radio 4 and *Rough Justice*.